Low Back Pain
and
Low Back Care

by Dr. Vinod A. Mittal
MS (Orth.), MBBS, DPC
Orthopedic Surge

Translators
Hindi: Priti V. Mittal
Spanish: Altagracia P. Ma,
Haitian Creole: Idi Jawarakim
Portuguese: Patricia B.P. Dos Santos

English–Hindi–Spanish–Haitian Creole–Portuguese

Trilingual Press
Cambridge, Massachusetts

Low Back Pain
and
Low Back Care

by Dr. Vinod A. Mittal

MS (Orth.), MBBS, DPC

Orthopedic Surgeon

English–Hindi–Spanish–Haitian Creole–Portuguese

Translators

Hindi: Priti V. Mittal

Spanish: Altagracia P. Mayers

Haitian Creole: Idi Jawarakim

Portuguese: Patricia B.P. Dos Santos

Graphic design

David Henry

ISBN 10: 0-9745821-7-4

ISBN 13: 978-0-9745821-7-7

Library of Congress Control Number: 2009940022

Published by Trilingual Press

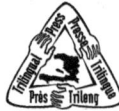

PO Box 391206

Cambridge, MA 02139

Tel. 617-331-2269

Email: trilingualpress@tanbou.com

First US edition September 2010

Foreword

Low back pain, with or without associated sciatica is one of the most common medical problems. In my days as an orthopedic resident medical officer in the 1970s, I was rather disappointed with the treatment of this condition. Conservative management consisted of bed rest, leg traction, medications and back extension exercises (backward bending). If there was inadequate relief in six weeks, a myelogram was done to find out if there was a neural compromise, and if so, an operation performed such as removal of the intervertebral disc. Many patients had temporary relief and then returned with low back pain and sciatica in a year or two. In one hospital's orthopedic unit where I took over as head of the unit in the 1980s, 40 of the 64 backs operated upon returned with low back pain and/or sciatica.

An alternative was sought and found in conservative (a specific type), non-operative management. The results of conservative treatment have been shown to be comparative or even superior to operative treatment. I have treated about 15,000 patients of low back pain with conservative management as outlined in this book with gratifying results.

This book is meant for educating the lay person as well as general medical practitioners and paramedicos.

The booklet in English has proven to be of value in imparting education on the subject. Subsequently it was brought out in Hindi and Marathi to reach out to more people in India where it has received much media coverage.

I am grateful to Eddy Toussaint, the publisher of the present book, for bringing this out in five languages to reach a still wider audience. Many thanks too to all the translators, Priti Mittal (also the illustrator), Altagracia P. Mayers, Patricia B.P. Dos Santos and Idi Jawarakim. Finally, thanks to family members Bharati, Nikhil and Ravi for technical help.

—Dr. Vinod A. Mittal

Index of Languages

Low Back Pain and Low Back Care

by Dr. Vinod A. Mittal
MS (Orth.), MBBS, DPC
Orthopedic Surgeon

Contents

Understanding of low back pain and sciatica

Low back pain (LBP) occurs in 80% to 97% of the adult population, disabling enough to prevent normal routine, as reported by different workers on the subject. It is the commonest cause of man-hours of work lost in industry.

The spine, developmentally, was never meant to take weight; but only to protect the spinal cord. However, it was forced to take upon the former function ever since man evolved from a quadruped to a biped. It would probably take millions of years for the spine to adapt itself to this new weight-bearing function.

Up to teenage years and even early childhood, the bones have a layer of cartilage, which, being resilient, acts as a buffer, absorbing shock of weight bearing, walking, running etc. By the age of 22 to 25 years, most of the cartilage is absorbed into relatively harder bone. Buffering action no longer occurs effectively and bone impacts against bone, causing inflammation in the joints, especially the weight bearing ones, adhesions, outgrowing of the ends etc., namely osteoarthrosis. The cumulative effect of this shows up as stiffness and pain.

Ageing cannot be prevented, but its effects can be decreased by low back care—something everyone should learn about just as much as say, dental care. However, before one proceeds to low back care, it is good to understand the mechanics of low back pain.

The spine if seen from front backwards is meant to be in a straight line (fig. 1). However, in many people, it might be curved. The vertebrae are the building blocks of the spine. In a curved spine, the inter-vertebral space opens up on the convex side and gets closer on the concave side as in a bent rod. This causes unevenness of pressures

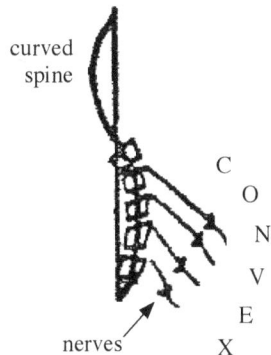

curved spine

CONVEX

nerves

Fig. 1

---

on the vertebral articulations, predisposing to osteoarthrosis. Note that, in between vertebrae, spinal nerves coming from the spinal cord, exit. These may get compromised, stretched or compressed, giving rise to pain radiating from the low back to the lower limbs, usually at the back of the limb, referred to as sciatica.

When viewed from the side, the

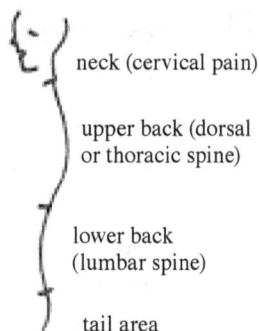

neck (cervical pain)

upper back (dorsal or thoracic spine)

lower back (lumbar spine)

tail area

Fig. 2

spine has natural forward and backward curves as shown (fig. 2).

The lower back is a forward curve and consists of five vertebrae (fig. 3). Each vertebra throws out a pair of upper and lower processes on either side of the midline. The lower processes of the upper vertebra articulate with the respective upper processes of the lower vertebra to form joints called facet joints. The facet joint is a lubricated joint and with constant rubbing of the joint surfaces predisposes to inflammation.

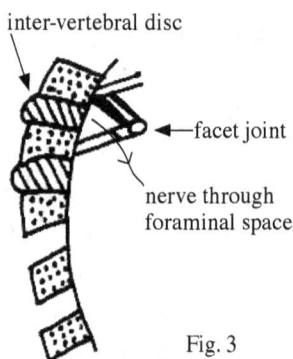

inter-vertebral disc

facet joint

nerve through foraminal space

Fig. 3

From the accompanying diagram, it is clear that if the facet joints become arthritic or if there is protrusion of the disc sandwiched between vertebrae, the exiting nerve roots in the foramen (hole) as shown may get compromised giving sciatica in addition to LBP.

The greater the depth of the forward curve, the greater the chances of inflammation in the facet joints. When such inflammation (I) occurs, it gives rise to pain (P), which causes spasm (S) of the muscles on either side of the spine (the spine is felt as a longitudinal groove in between two longitudinal bulges on either side formed by the muscles) which gives further pain (fig. 4).

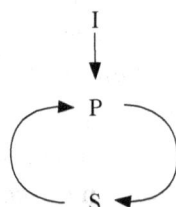

I

P

S

Fig. 4

Low Back Pain and Low Back Care

Thus a vicious cycle is set up which can manifest as chronic, grumbling LBP, with or without acute exacerbations and radiation to lower limbs.

What increases the normal forward curvature of the lumbar spine? (fig. 5).

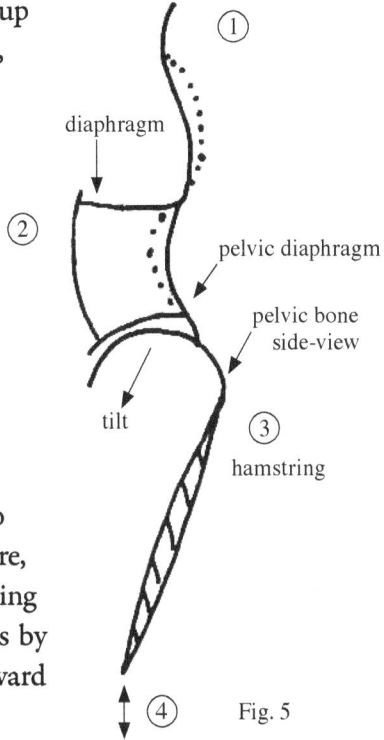

Fig. 5

1. **An increased backward curve**, a hump, of the upper back (shown by dotted lines in the figure).

2. **Abdominal bulge** due to weak abdominal musculature, a paunch, pregnancy, carrying of weights in the front as by librarians, will cause a forward drag on the low back.

3. **Tight hamstring muscles:** These muscles are attached from the back of the pelvis to the back of the knee. If tight, they cause a tilting of the pelvis to which the spine is attached and a consequent increased forward bend.

4. **High heels:** It is common knowledge that high heels produce a strutted gait. This is because the pelvis is tilted forwards from above and carries with it the lower spine.

Many other conditions can also cause LBP (e.g. infections) and sciatica (e.g. diabetes). These are not being dealt with in this article which concentrates on the usual mechanical LBP. Also, mental and emotional stresses are known to cause pain in the spine. This is due to a state of chronic tensed muscle and a symbolic translation of carrying a "load" on the back or keeping problems behind one as it were.

Low back care

Having understood the "why" of low back pain (LBP), the "how" of low back care becomes easy to follow. However, one could proceed to do this even without understanding the mechanics of LBP.

One has to be realistic in expectations. Since total prevention of chronological ageing of the spine is not possible, one can only retard it and its effects. Hence one would prevent pain relatively, or decrease its amplitude and frequency (fig. 6).

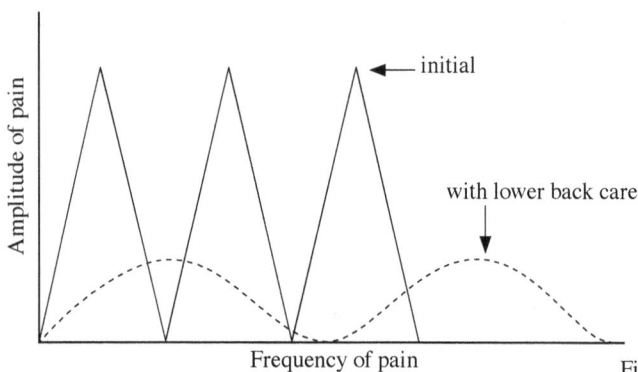

Fig. 6

If the lumbar spine is unbalanced, curved, as viewed from front backwards or vice-versa, it is simply corrected by raising the footwear on the convex side of the curve. To see imbalances for yourself, stand in under-clothes with feet together, upper limbs hanging down, in front of a tall mirror. There is a natural gap between the elbows and waist. This is equal in a straight spine, but decreased on the convex side with increase on the concave side in a curved spine. To balance this, keep increasing the footwear by 1 cm. each time on the convex side (one can use wooden planks or footwear with different sized heels) till the gap is equal. This can be confirmed by having another person or doctor viewing the spine from the back.

Obliteration of the increased forward curve of the lumbar spine would involve tightening the abdominal musculature, loosening the hamstrings, stretching the paraspinal muscles spanning the spine to relieve spasm, and doing away with or reducing high heels if any, especially during pain episodes. Half to three-fourth inch heels might be alright. If one wants additional height, it is best to use a platform raise.

The vicious cycle of inflammation, pain, spasm, needs to be broken by use of posture, exercises, heat, medications, and surgery (which is not being dealt with). Most LBPs can be dealt with by conservative means.

Medications would be of the anti-inflammatory group primarily, supplemented if necessary with painkillers. Medications are best taken with food and antacids to prevent irritation of the stomach lining.

Heat, short of short wave diathermy given by a physiotherapist, can be applied at home by means of hot, wet, towel application. Cover the back with it, cover over with plastic to retain moisture and heat. When pain decreases with muscle relaxation, use the opportunity to practice exercises. Note that infra-red lamps do not provide penetrating heat and as such are useless.

Posture

Sitting: One should not sit on the chair right at the back, as usually taught, which will increase the forward curve of the lumbar spine. Sit somewhat in the front, with knees raised, allowing the low back to slouch. One could cross the ankle or knee over the opposite knee (fig. 7). While sitting at a table, pull the chair close to the table and use the foot-bar which should be close to your side of the table (fig. 8). If there is no bar, use a box or draw

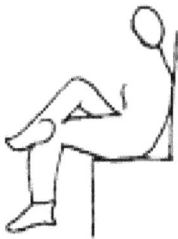

Fig. 7

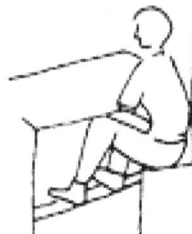

Fig. 8

to rest the feet. The idea is to raise the knees, if possible higher than the hips, thereby tilting the pelvis forward from below and pushing the low back backwards. At home one could choose to sit on a low surface (fig. 9) so that the knees are automatically high or sit atop any surface with feet on it (fig. 10).

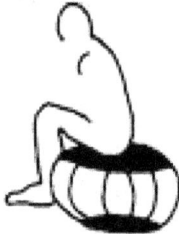 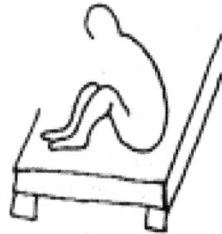

Fig. 9   Fig. 10

While in a road vehicle however, sit at the back of the seat and use a small pillow to fill up the gap between the lower spine and back rest. This will help in absorption of the vertical shocks through the spine. If driving, in addition to the above, keep your seat comfortably close to the foot-panels so that the knees are sufficiently elevated.

Lying down: On a wooden surface use a firm mattress. A thick, cotton one is the best. The spine can now be adjusted against it. Hard ground is unnecessary and hurts the bony prominences.

A soft mattress does not allow adaptation of the spine against it. Prone lying, on the stomach, is to be avoided since the low back remains backward bent with a forward curve. If lying on the back, bend knees, feet flat on the bed, and use a bolster or two pillows under the knees for support. This posture flattens the lumbar spine against the bed (fig. 11). If side-lying (left is more comfortable if sleeping on a heavy stomach which receives support), the

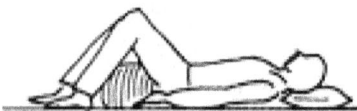

Fig. 11

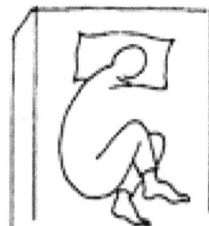

Fig. 12

hips and knees are bent, pulled up towards the chest, one may be more than the other (fig. 12).

Standing: Intermittently, consciously sitting or bending forward and springing, when possible, takes a lot of strain off the spine. When standing straight on both feet, the pelvis remains in a locked position. Intermittent unlocking, by slightly bending one knee and mildly swaying the pelvis to the opposite side helps (fig. 13).

Working in a standing position, as in cooking, ironing etc. can be very demolishing for the low back. The do's and dont's are shown (fig. 14).

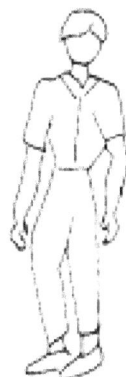

Fig. 13

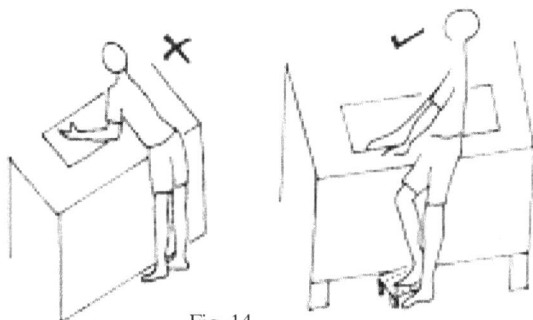

Fig. 14

Keep the work surface and body close to each other. Space below the work surface, for the feet, helps. Use a foot stool under one foot and keep alternating from foot to foot at intervals of time.

Walking: Again, intermittently sitting or bending forward and springing is very good.

Lifting weights: The spine is at its weakest in a forward, bent position. Imagine children's play blocks placed exactly vertically over each other. A knock from the top does not topple them. However, if placed in a curved fashion, they would easily fall when knocked.

When weights are carried from the front with lower limbs straight more or less and spine bent forward, the fulcrum is in the spine and the weight far away thus giving no mechanical advantage and thereby straining the back. Whenever possible, keep the

weight close on the side.
Bend the lower limbs, keep
the spine relatively straight
and use the thigh muscles
to help lift the weight as one
straightens the lower limbs
(fig. 15).

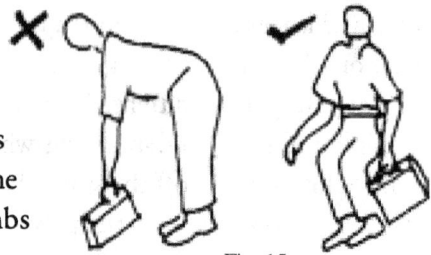

Fig. 15

Exercises

These along with posture form the mainstay of low back care. The exercises are meant to stretch the paraspinal spasmodic muscles, tighten the abdominal musculature, loosen the hamstrings, break adhesions in the synovial joints and help self-manipulation of the spine.

Standing exercises:

1. **Toe-touching:** Feet near together. Try to touch the toes by bending forward. Do not bend from the hips and reach down. Take care to bend the

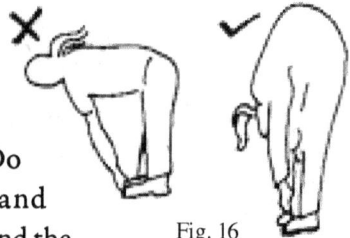

Fig. 16

spine by keeping the head close to the body and rolling the vertebrae one over the other (fig. 16). Reaching the toes or ground is not important but doing the maximum one can. Avoid gross jerky forward bending. Springing is however good. Breathing out helps as one bends down.

2. **Twist and jerk:** Feet apart one to 1.5 ft., hands on hips, twist maximum to the left (fig. 17). Then slightly derotate and gently jerk to maximum again. Jerk twice. Then back to neutral position. Now twist and repeat the manoeuvre to the right. If one has knee problems, this exercise is best done in a sitting position at the edge of an armless chair or bed. This will avoid twisting at the knee.

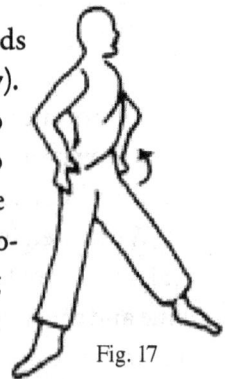

Fig. 17

3. **Cross toe-touch:** Feet wide apart. With the right hand fingers try and cross over to reach the left toes (fig. 18). Come up to neutral. Then vice-versa.

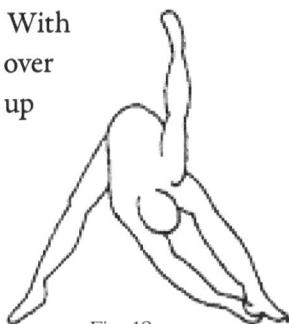

Fig. 18

4. **Alternate toe-heel-touch:** Feet wide apart. With the left hand fingers, attempt to touch the toes of the same side. To neutral. Now try to reach with the right hand fingers the right heel (fig. 19). To neutral. Then vice-versa.

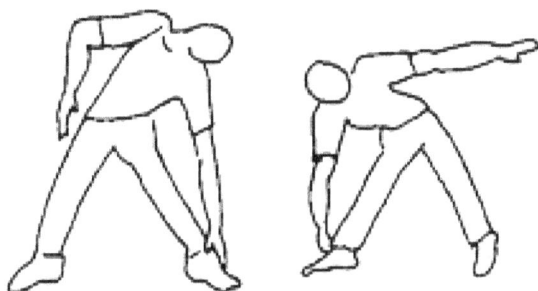

Fig. 19

5. **Side-bending:** Feet wide apart. Upper limbs outstretched on the sides. Bend sideways to left taking the left upper limb along the leg. Stretch the right upper limb upwards and look towards it (fig. 20). To neutral. Repeat to the right side.

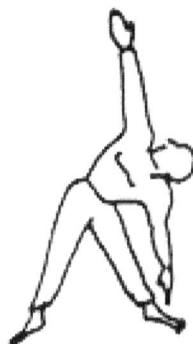

Fig. 20

6. **Kick:** Take one or two steps forward and swing the left lower limb straight up to touch the fingers of the outstretched left upper limb held at about shoulder height (fig. 21). Take care not to slip and fall backwards by avoiding slippery ground or footwear. Then repeat with the right side.

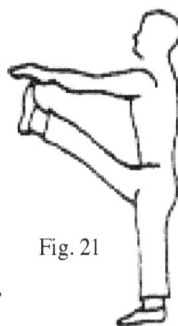

Fig. 21

Lying down exercises:

(on a firm or hard surface e.g. groundsheet on the floor)

7. Hands behind head. Feet together. Outstretched lower limbs. Breathe in, hold. Raise feet a few inches till there is maximum strain in the midline of the abdomen, hold to a count of ten (this may require building up to ten over some time), then lower (fig. 22).

8. Repeat the above with feet wide apart. The strain is mainly felt in the lower and outer part of the abdomen.

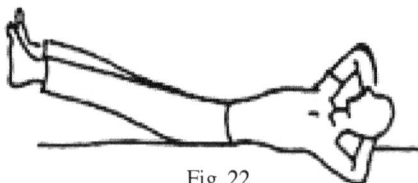

Fig. 22

9. Lie flat on the back, arms on the side. Bend the left hip and knee and clasp just below the knee with hands. Bring the knee towards the right shoulder which can be arched forwards. Keep the right lower limb straight (fig. 23). Exhalation helps. Repeat with the opposite sides.

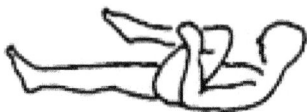

Fig. 23

10. Lie flat, arms outstretched above and behind the head. Get up and try and reach the toes (fig. 24). Breathing out helps. If you cannot get up, ask someone to hold the legs down, or hook your toes under heavy furniture, say a cupboard, to help you. If you cannot reach the toes, grasp whatever part of the leg you can reach and pull yourself down attempting to bury your head between the lower limbs.

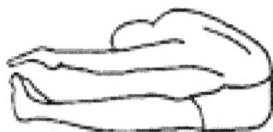

Fig. 24

All of the above exercises are to be done three times each. It takes about 7 minutes. Once a day is usually enough. Twice is recommended when there is pain.

Note that forward bending of the spine is known to increase the spinal canal space in the vertebrae, through which the spinal cord descends from the brain. It also increases the foraminal space thus taking pressure off the nerves. This is an additional benefit in neural radiating pain.

A word of caution. Many other conditions can also give rise to LBP or sciatica. These need to be ruled out by simple investigations, most often blood tests and x-rays. However, most backaches fall under the category of a strain phenomenon and can be taken care of by low back care.

Finally, psychological stresses need to be taken care of by learning relaxation techniques and understanding the art of living.

Disclaimer

The material in this book is intended for most mechanical low back pains and not for infections, tumors, etc. Please consult a physician for establishing the cause of the low back pain. The author, translators and publisher are not responsible for any damage that might arise from the utilisation of the contents of this book.

पीठ का दर्द
और
पीठ की देखभाल

डॉ. वि. अ. मित्तल

एम. एस. (अस्थिव्यंग)
एम. बी. बी. एस.
डी. पी. सी.

अस्थिव्यंग शल्यचिकित्सक

अनुवादक : प्रीती वि. मित्तल

विषय

Low Back Pain and Low Back Care

पीठ के निचले हिस्से का दर्द और शियाटिका का ग्यान

रीढ़ के निचले हिस्से का दर्द ८०-९६% प्रौढ़ लोगों में होता है , जिससे उन्हें रोजमर्रा के कामकाज में परेशानी होती है । ऐसा इस विषय पर कार्य करने वाले जानकारों का मत है । यह एक मुख्य कारण है जिसकी वजह से औद्यौगिक संस्थाओं में कामकाज के घंटे खोये जाते है ।

रीढ़ की हड्डी का मुख्य कार्य सिर्फ मेरुदंड की हिफाज़त करना था, न कि बोझ उठाने का काम । लेकिन जब से मानव ने चार पैरों वाले प्राणी से दो पैरों वाले प्राणी तक की प्रगति की , उसे मज़बूरन यह कार्य करना पड़ा । इस ढाँचे को शायद हज़ारों वर्ष लग जायेंगे, जब वह इस बोझ उठाने वाली नई भूमिका को निभाने मे समर्थ होगा ।

युवा अवस्था और उसके कुछ समय बाद तक हड्डियों पर एक तह कार्टिलेज की होती है । यह लचीला होने की वजह से शरीर पर पड़ने वाले किसी भी प्रकार के धक्के को सह लेने वाले मध्यस्थ (बफ्फर) का काम करती है । बोझ उठाने, दौड़ने, चलने आदि गतिविधियों से उत्पन्न कम्पन को सहने में मदद करती है । लेकिन उम्र के २०-२५ वर्ष तक यह कार्टिलेज सख्त हड्डियों के रूप में परिवर्तित हो जाती है । धक्के को सहन करने की शक्ति कम हो जाती है । एक हड्डी दूसरे हड्डी से टकराती है जिससे जोड़ों में सूजन और चिपचिपाहट हो जाती है, खासकर वज़न उठाने वाले जोड़ों मे इनके छोर बढ़ जाते है । इस स्थिति को औस्टिओ-आर्थोसिस कहते है। इससे जोड़ों में दर्द और कड़ापन आ जाता ह ।

उम्र के बढ़न को तो रोका नहीं जा सकता , लेकिन उनके कारण होने वाले प्रभावों को पीठ की देखभाल से कम अवश्य किया जा सकता है । हरएक को इसका ग्यान होना उतना ही ज़रूरी है , जितना कि दाँतों की देखभाल का ग्यान होना । बहरहाल , पीठ के निचले भाग की देखभाल की जानकारी प्राप्त करने से पहले यह समझना आवश्यक है कि यह दर्द किस प्रकार उत्पन्न होता है ।

रीढ़ को आगे से पीछे की ओर देखने से इसे एक सरल रेखा में होना चाहिये, लेकिन कुछ लोगों में यह टेढ़ा या कमानाकार होता है (आकृति १) । मेरूदंड अलग अलग जोड़ों या मनकों (vertebrae) से बना एक ढाँचा है। कमानाकार मेरूदंड में इन जोड़ों के मध्य का भाग बाहर की ओर (convex) खुलता है और धसा हुआ (concave) भाग नज़दीक आता है जिस तरह मुड़े हुए सलिये में होता है । इससे रीढ़ की हड्डी पर असमतल दबाव पड़ता है , जिसके कारण औस्टिओ-आर्थोसिस

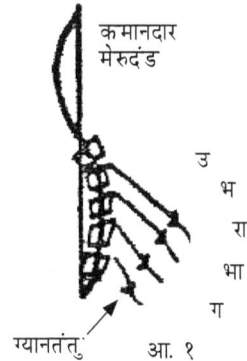

कमानदार मेरूदंड

उभराभाग

ग्यानतंतु

आ. १

हो सकता है। मनकों के बीच में, मेरूदंड से निकले ग्यानतंतु (nerves) होते है। इन पर दबाव या खिंचाव पड़ सकता है। इसके कारण रीढ़ के निचले , और टाँगों के पिछले भाग से ऐड़ी तक दर्द का संचार हो सकता है । इसे शियाटिका कहते हैं ।

शरीर को अगर दायें या बायें ओर से देखें तो रीढ़ में प्राकृतिक रूप से सामने और पीछे की ओर कमानाकार दिखाई देगा जैसा कि आ. २ मे दिखाई गया है ।

रीढ़ के निचले भाग में सामने की ओर कक्का (curve) होता है। इसमें पाँच मनके होते है (आ. ३) । हर जोड़ के पिछले भाग से दायें और बायें तरफ एक जोड़ हड्डियों का उभार होता है । ऊपरी जोड़ का निचला उभार, निचले जोड़ के ऊपरी उभार से मिलकर एक संधि (joint) बनता है जिसे फेसेट (facet joint) जौईंट कहते है ।

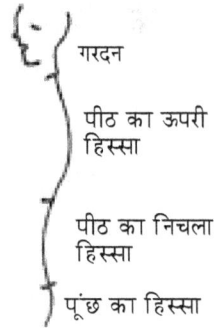

गरदन
पीठ का ऊपरी हिस्सा
पीठ का निचला हिस्सा
पूंछ का हिस्सा

आ. २

यह जौईंट चिकना या स्निग्ध होता है ,लेकिन बार–बार के घर्षण से जौईंट सतह पर सूजन आ सकती है । प्रस्तुत चित्र को (आ.३) देखने से यह ज़ाहिर हो सकता है कि अगर फैसिट जौईंट में संधिवात (arthritis) हो जाये या दो जोड़ो के बीच की गद्दी (disc) पीछे की तरफ खिसक जाये, तो छिद्र से निकलने वाले ग्यानतंतु दब सकते है । इसके कारण रीढ़ के निचले भाग के साथ–साथ शियाटिका का दर्द भी हो सकता है ।

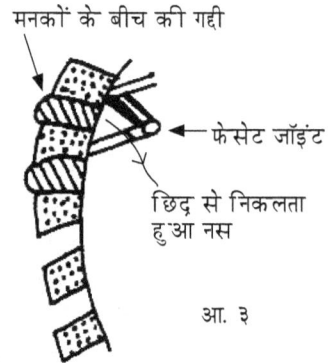

मनकों के बीच की गद्दी

फेसेट जॉइंट

छिद्र से निकलता हुआ नस

आ. ३

रीढ़ की हड्डी में सामने का कमानाकार जितना गहरा होगा , फेसेट जौईंट में सूजन होने का खतरा उतना ही अधिक होगा । इससे दर्द बढ़ता है और तीव्र पीडा से मेरूदंड के दोनों तरफ के माँसपेशियों में ऐंठन पैदा होता है, जिससे दर्द और भी बढ़ता है (आ. ४) । इस तरह एक खतरनाक चक्र स्थापित हो जाता है, जो स्थायी रूप से रीढ़ के निचले भागों में दर्द बनाये रखता है । यह दर्द कभी– कभी अधिक तीव्र हो सकता है या शियाटिका के रूप में आ सकता है।

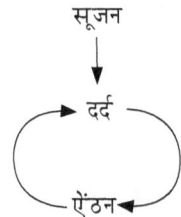

सूजन

दर्द

ऐंठन

आ. ४

रीढ़ के सामान्य कमानाकार में अधिक गहराई आने का कारण क्या है ? (आ. ५)

१. **पीठ के ऊपरी भाग के कमानाकार मे बढ़ोत्तरी** (चित्र में बिन्दुओं के द्वारा दर्शाया गया है) ।

२. **पेट का मोटापन**: यह पेट के कमज़ोर माँसपेशियों के कारण, तोंद निकलने गर्भावस्था या सामने से वज़न उठाने से जैसे कि लाईब्रेरियन करते है ; इनके कारण होता है । इसमें रीढ़ के निचले भाग को सामने की ओर खिंचाव मिलता है ।

३. **हैमस्ट्रिंग (Hamstring) माँसपेशियों में तनाव:** ये माँसपेशियाँ पैल्विस (pelvis) के पिछले भाग से घुटनों के पिछले भाग तक जुड़ी होती हैं । इसमें तनाव होने से यह पैल्विस को एक तरह झुका देती है । पैल्विस रीढ़ की हड्डी के साथ जुड़ा रहता है, परिणाम स्वरूप रीढ़ की हड्डी का झुकाव सामने की ओर बढ़ जाता है ।

४. **ऊँची एड़ी के जूते:** सभी जानते है कि ऊँची एड़ियों से चाल में अकड़पन आ जाता है । इसका कारण यह है कि पैल्विस ऊपर से आगे की ओर जाता है और अपने साथ रीढ़ के निचले भाग के कमानाकार को आगे बढ़ा देता है ।

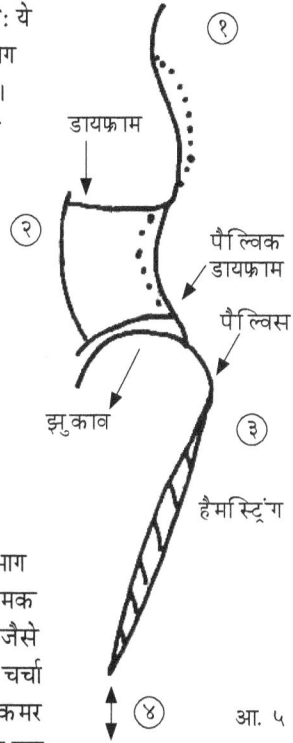

आ. ५

और भी कई कारण है जो कमर के निचले भाग में दर्द पैदा कर सकते हैं जैसे कि रीढ़ में संक्रामक रोग । शियाटिका भी अन्य कारणों से हो सकता है जैसे कि मधुमेह में । इस लेख में इन समस्याओं की चर्चा नहीं की जा रही है ; बल्कि यहाँ आम यांत्रिक कमर के निचले भाग के दर्द की ओर ध्यान केंद्रित किया गया है । इसके अलावा देखा गया है कि मानसिक और भावनात्मक दबाव भी कमर के दर्द का कारण बन सकते है । ऐसा इसलिये होता है कि लंबे अरसे तक माँसपेशियाँ तनाव की स्थिति में रहती है और मानसिक रूप से मानो समस्याओं के बोझ को पीठ पर ढोते रहने से या समस्याओं को पीछे धकेलते रहने से,यह स्थिति उत्पन्न होती है ।

पीठ की देखभाल

शरीर के पृष्ठ भाग में दर्द 'क्यों' होता है, यह जानने के बाद, उसकी देखभाल किस प्रकार करनी चाहिये, यह समझना आसान हो जाता है। यह किस प्रकार होता है, इस कार्य प्रणाली को जानना आवश्यक नहीं है।

हमें थोड़ा यथार्थवादी होना चाहिये, क्योंकि आयु के साथ-साथ रीढ़ की हड्डी का कमज़ोर होना तो रोका नहीं जा सकता। किन्तु हम इसके परिणाओं को मंद अवश्य कर सकते है। इस तरह पीड़ा को एक हद तक रोका या उसकी तीव्रता और रफ्तार को कम किया जा सकता है (आ. ६)।

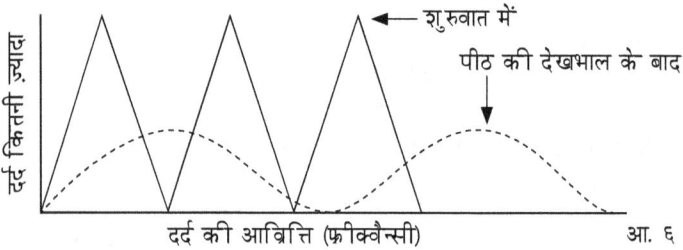

दर्द की आवृत्ति (फ्रीक्वैन्सी)   आ. ६

अगर रीढ़ के कमर के भाग को सामने से पीछे की ओर या पीछे से सामने की ओर देखने से वह असंतुलित कमानदार दिखाई दे, तो इसे आसानी से जूते के बाहरी उभार को ऊँचा करके सुधारा जा सकता है। इस संतुलन को स्वयं देखना हो तो, बड़े शीशे के सामने दोनों एड़ियों को जोड़कर, दोनों बाज़ुओं को ढीला छोड़कर, खड़े हो जायें। आप देखेंगे कि कुहनी और कमर के बीच एक रिक्त स्थान रहता है। सीधी रीढ़ वालों में यह एक समान होता है, जब कि कमानाकार रीढ़ की हड्डी वालों में यह बाहर की तरफ (convex) में कम और अंदर की ओर अधिक होता है। इस संतुलन को बनाये रखने के लिये जूते को बाहर की ओर (concave) एक सेमी. (cm.) बढ़ाते रहना चाहिये (चाहे तो लकड़ी के पट्टे का इस्तेमाल कर सकते है, या अलग–अलग नाप की एड़ियों के जूते पहन सकते है) जबतक कमर और कुहनी के बीच का अंतर बराबर न हो जाये। इसे देखने के लिये आप किसी अन्य व्यक्ति या डॉक्टर को कह सकते हैं।

रीढ़ की हड्डी को कमर के भाग में सामने की ओर बढ़े हुए कमानाकार को समाप्त करने के लिये पेट की माँसपेशियों का कसना, हैमस्ट्रिंग माँसपेशियों को ढीला करना, रीढ़ के दोनों तरफ के ऐंठे हुए माँसपेशियों में खिंचाव लाना, और ऊँची एड़ियों के जूते पहनना ज़रूरत पड़ने पर खासकर दर्द की स्थिति में, आवश्यक है। आधे से पौने इंच की एड़ी पहनने में हर्ज नहीं है। यदि कोई कद की अधिक ऊँचाई चाहें तो बेहतर होगा कि वह पूरे तलुवे की समांतर ऊँचाई बढ़ायें (platform sole)।

सूजन (inflammation) के साथ दर्द, ऐंठन आदि का कुचक्र तोड़ने के लिये सही आसन, व्यायाम, दवाईयाँ, सेक और शल्य चिकित्सा (इसकी चर्चा इस

लेख में नहीं की जा रही है) का सहारा लिया जा सकता है। अधिकतर कमर का दर्द रूढ़िवादि या साधारण तरीकों द्वारा कम किया जा सकता है ।

दवाईयाँ : ये मुख्यतः सूजन को कम करने वाले वर्ग की होंगी, आवश्यकता पड़ने पर साथमें दर्दनाशक दवाईयाँ भी दी जा सकती है । इन दवाईयों को भोजन के साथ लेना सबसे उत्तम होगा और साथ में आम्लनाशक औषधी (antacids) का सेवन करना चाहिये ताकि पेट की परत मे जलन ना हो ।

सेंक : गरम किरणों का उपचार फिज़ियो–थेरापिस्ट देते हैं जिसे short wave diathermy कहते है । घर पर गरम गीले तौलिये का सेंक दिया जा सकता है। गरम पानी में तौलिये को डुबाकर निचोड़ लें इससे पीठ को ढक दें। उष्णता और नमी को अधिक समय तक बरकरार रखने के लिये उसपर प्लस्टिक बिछा दें । जब माँसपेशीयों को राहत मिलेगी और दर्द कम होगा , यह मौका व्यायाम करने में लगायें। इस बात की नोद लें कि लाल किरणों वाली बत्तियाँ (infra red lamps) शरीर के भीतर प्रवेश कर सेंक नहीं दे सकती , इसलिये इलाज के लिये निरूपयोगी है ।

मुद्रा या आसन

बैठना : कुर्सी पर बिल्कुल पीछे की ओर सटकर नहीं बैठना चाहिये जैसा कि साधारणतः सिखाया जाता है। इससे मेरूदंड का निचला भाग सामने की ओर अधिक कमानाकार हो जायेगा। कुर्सी पर कुछ आगे खिसककर बैठें , घुटनों को थोड़ा ऊपर रखें ताकि कमर का हिस्सा विश्राम की स्थिति में रहे । चाहें तो एक टाँग के घुटने या एड़ी को दूसरी टाँग के घुटने पर रखकर बैठें (आ. ७)। कुर्सी को टेबल के बिलकुल नज़दीक खेचकर बैठें। पैर रखने वाली पट्टी पर पैरों को टिकायें। यह पट्टी आपके करीब होनी चाहिये (आ. ८)। अगर पैरों को टिकाने के लिये कोई पट्टी न हो तो किसी बक्से या दराज़ का इस्तेमाल करें । इसका उद्देश्य केवल घुटनों की सतह को ऊपर उठाना है, अगर संभव हो तो कमर की सतह से ऊँचा । इससे पैल्विस का झुकाव नीचे से आगे की ओर होगा और कमर के निचले हिस्से को पीछे की ओर दबाव मिलेगा ।

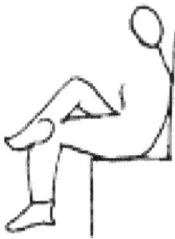 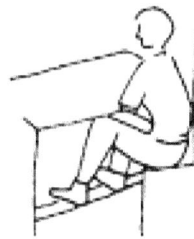

आ. ७   आ. ८

घर पर हम अपनी इच्छानुसार बैठने के लिये निचली सतह चुन सकते है (आ. ९) जिससे अपने आप घुटने ऊपर की ओर रहेंगे। पलंग या दीवान पर पैर ऊपर रखकर बैठ सकते है (आ. १०) ।

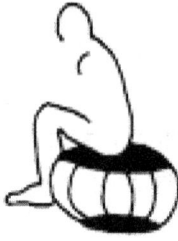
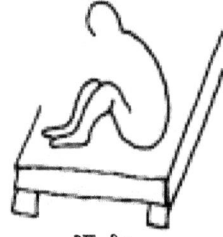

आ. ९   आ. १०

अगर आप सड़क पर किसी गाड़ी से यात्रा कर रहे हों , तो सीट के पिछले हिस्से से सटकर बैठें लेकिन कमर के निचले हिस्से में एक छोटा तकिया रख लें , जिससे रीढ़ मे लगने वाले आकस्मिक धक्के का कम असर होगा। गाड़ी चलाते समय ऊपरी बताये हिदायतों के अलावा , अपनी सीट को ब्रेक-क्लच के जितना नज़दीक रख सकते है रखें, ताकि घुटने किसी हद तक ऊपर की ओर उठे रहें ।

लेटना : लेटने के लिये लकड़ी की सतह पर सख्त गद्दों का इस्तेमाल करें क्योंकि रीढ़ की हड्डी को गद्दी की ओर दबाया जा सकता है । रुई का गद्दा सबसे आम होता है। सख्त ज़मीन पर लेटना अनावश्यक है क्योंकि इससे हड्डियों के उभरे भागों में पीड़ा ही होगी । नरम गद्दे पीठ के कमानाकार रिक्त स्थान में भर जाते है और इसे सीधे नहीं होने देते । पेट के बल लेटना हितकारी नहीं होगा क्योंकि इससे कमर का निचला हिस्सा पीछे की ओर मुड़ा रहता है और सामने की ओर कमानाकार बनाता है । पीठ के बल लेटे हो तो घुटनों को मोड़ लें , तलुवों को बिस्तर पर सपाट रखें , और घुटनों के नीचे गोल गद्दा या दो तकिये सहारे के लिये रखें। इस मुद्रा में कमर का निचला हिस्सा बिस्तर पर सपाट रहता है (आ. ११) ।

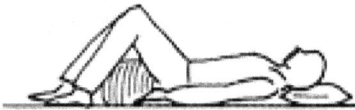
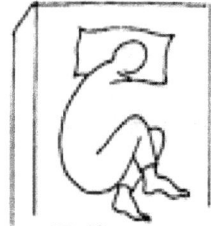

आ. ११   आ. १२

अगर एक करवट पर लेटना हो (भोजन के बाद आराम से बाईं करवट पर लेटने से पेट को सहारा मिलता है) तो कुल्हों और घुटनों को मोड़कर छाती की ओर खींच लें । एक घुटना दूसरे घुटने के मुकाबले छाती के ज़्यादा करीब हो सकता है (आ. १२) ।

खड़े रहना : हमें सचेत होना पड़ेगा कि लगातार सीधे खड़े होने की बजाय थोड़ी थोड़ी देर में कभी बैठें , आगे झुकें और स्प्रिंग की तरह रीढ़ की हड्डी को ऊपर नीचे करें । दोनो टाँगों पर अधिक समय तक सीधे खड़े रहने से पैल्विस कमर के निचले भाग को जकड़ देती है । इस जकड़न से छुटकारा पाने के लिये एक घुटने

को थोड़ा सा मोड़ना चाहिये , ऐसा करने से रीढ़ का तनाव कम हो जाता है । बीच-बीच में एक घुटने को थोड़ा मोड़ने और पैल्विस को विपरित दिशा में घुमाने से मदद मिल सकती है (आ. १३) ।

खड़े होकर काम करना जैसे खाना बनाना , कपड़ों पर इस्त्री करना , आदि , कमर के निचले भाग के लिये काफ़ी कष्टदायक हो सकता है । सही और गलत तरीकों की जानकारी आकृति १४ में दी गई है । काम करने वाली सतह शरीर के करीब होनी चाहिये । काम की सतह के नीचे , पैर रखने के लिये पर्याप्त जगह होनी चाहिये । पैर के नीचे एक छोटा स्टूल रख लें जो कि अदल-बदल कर कभी दायें कभी बायें पैर के नीचे रख सकते है । इससे आराम मिलेगा ।

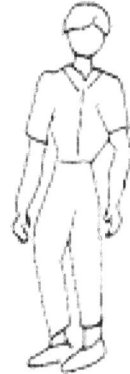

आ. १३

चलना : फिर से वही थोड़ी-थोड़ी देर में बैठने , आगे की ओर मुड़ने और स्प्रिंग की तरह ऊपर नीचे होने से फायदा होगा ।

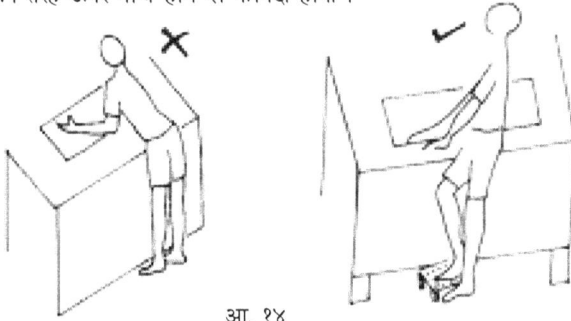

आ. १४

वज़न उठाना : रीढ़ के हड्डी जब सामने की ओर झुकी हों तब वह कमज़ोर स्थिति में होती है । कल्पना कीजिये बच्चों के खेलने वाले लकड़ी के चौकोर (blocks) बिल्कुल सीधे में एक के ऊपर एक रखे है , अगर ऊपर से उसपर थपकी मारी जाये तो ये नहीं गिरेंगे । लेकिन इनके टेढ़ी रचना की जाये तो एक थपकी में आसानी से ढह जायेंगे । सामने से वज़न उठाने के लिये , टाँगो को तकरीबन सीधा रखकर पीठ की हड्डी को सामने की ओर झुकाया जाये , तब आधार या fulcrum रीढ़ में होता है और वज़न दूर । इससे वज़न उठाने में कोई यांत्रिक सहायता नहीं मिलती जिसकी वजह से पीठ पर तनाव या ज़ोर पड़ता है जब कभी संभव हो वज़न को शरीर के करीब रखें , घुटनों को मोड़ें , रीढ़ को जितना हो सके सीधा रखें और जाँघों की माँसपेशियों की मदद से वज़न उठाते हुए टाँगों को सीधा करें (आ. १५) ।

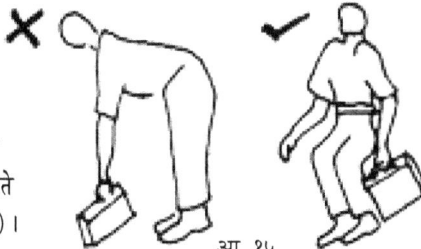

आ. १५

व्यायाम

पीठ की देखभाल में आसन और व्यायाम सबसे आवश्यक अंग है । व्यायाम का मकसद रीढ़ की हड्डी की आस-पास की माँसपेशियों में खिंचाव लाना, पेट की माँसपेशियों को तन कर रखना, हैमस्ट्रिंग पेशियों को ढीला करना और फैसेट जोड़ों में चिपचिपेपन को छुड़ाना है, तथा रीढ़ की हड्डी को आसानी से हलचल करने में मदद करना है ।

खड़े होकर करने वाले व्यायाम

१ **पैरों के अंगूठे को छूना :** दोनो पैरों को तकरीबन एक साथ रखें । आगे झुककर हाथों की ऊँगलियों को छूने का प्रयत्न करें । कुल्हों से मुड़कर नीचे न झुकें बल्कि ध्यान से रीढ़ की हड्डी को मोड़ें । ऐसा करने के लिये सिर को शरीर के करीब रखें और मेरूदंड के मनकों को एक के ऊपर एक लुढकते हुए नीचे झुकें (आ. १६) । पैरों की ऊँगलियों को या ज़मीन को छूना उतना ज़रूरी नहीं है जितना ऐसा करने का पूरा प्रयत्न करना । सामने झुकते वक्त बेमतलब ज़ोर से झटका न दें बल्कि स्प्रिंग की तरह ऊपर नीचे होना शरीर के लिये अच्छा है । नीचे झुकते वक्त श्वास छोड़ना सहायक सिद्ध होगा ।

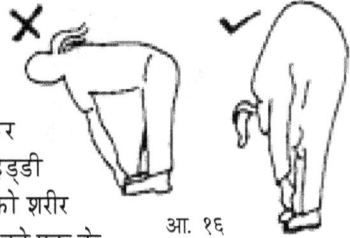

आ. १६

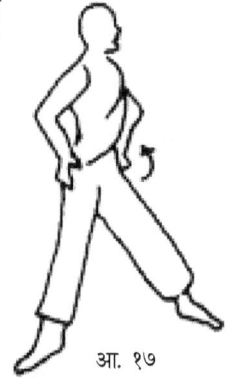

आ. १७

२ **ऐंठन और झटका :** टाँगों को १-१५ फुट की दूरी पर रखें । हाथ को कमर पर रखकर बाईं ओर जितना अधिक मुड़ सकते हैं मुड़ें (आ. १७) । फिर घूमकर थोड़ा पहली की स्थिति की ओर आयें और धीरे से झटका देकर फिर बाईं ओर मुड़ जायें, दो बार झटका दें । फिर पूर्व स्थिति में आ जायें । इसी कसरत को दाईं ओर से दोहरायें । किसी को अगर घुटने की तकलीफ है तो बेहतर होगा कि वह इसे बैठकर करे । इसे करने के लिये बिना बाज़ूवाले कुर्सी या पलंग छोर पर बैठना चाहिये । इससे घुटनों में ऐंठन नहीं होगी ।

३. **विपरीत पैरों के अंगूठे को छूना :** टाँगों को फैलाकर सीधे खड़े रहें । दायें हाथ की ऊँगलियों से झुककर बायें पैर की ऊँगलियों को छूने का प्रयत्न करें (आ. १८) । पूर्व स्थिति में लौट आयें । फिर बायें हाथ से इसी व्यायाम को दोहरायें ।

४. **पैरों के अंगूठे और एड़ी को बारी-बारी से छूना :** पैरों को दूर फैलाकर रखें । बायें हाथ की ऊँगलियों से बायें पैर की ऊँगलियो को छूने का प्रयास करें ।

पूर्व स्थिति में लौटें । अब दायें हाथ से दायें एड़ी को छूने की कोशिश करें (आ. १९) । पूर्व स्थिति में लौटें। अब इसे विपरीत हाथ से दोहरायें ।

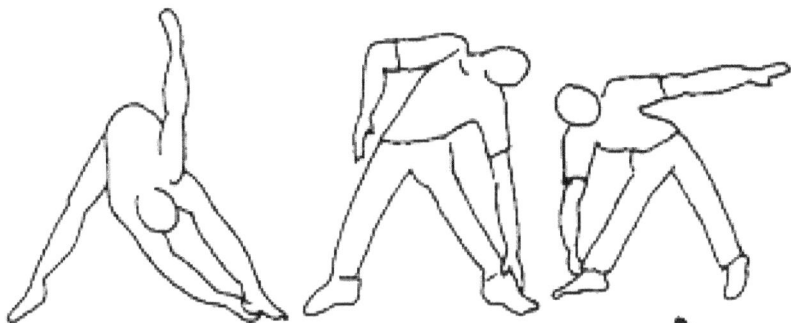

आ. १८   आ. १९

५. एक तरफा झुकाव : टाँगों को फैलाकर खड़े रहें । बाज़ुओं को दोनो तरफ फैलाकर रखें । बायें बाज़ू को बाईं तरफ टाँगो की सीध में झुकायें । दाहिनी बाँह को ऊपर सीधा रखें और नज़र वहीं घुमायें (आ. २०) । सामान्य स्थिति में लौटें । यही व्यायाम दायें हाथ से दोहरायें ।

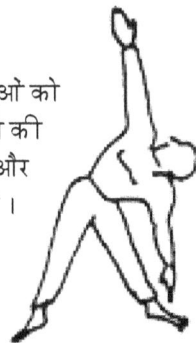

आ. २०

६. लात चलाना : एक दो कदम आगे बढ़ कर बायें पैर को सीधे ऊपर उठाकर बायें हाथ की ऊँगलियों से छूएं । बायाँ हाथ कंधे की ऊँचाई में होना चाहिये (आ. २१) । सावधानी बरतनी चाहिये ताकि आप फिसलकर पीठ के बल गिर न पड़ें । फिसलने वाले जूते और फिसलन वाली ज़मीन से दूर रहें । इसी कसरत को दाहिने टाँग में दोहरायें ।

लेटकर करने वाले व्यायाम : (इन्हें समतल सख्त सतह जैसे ज़मीन पर दरी बिछाकर करें)

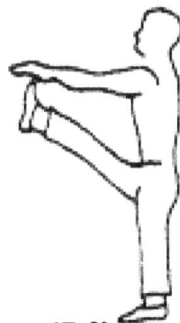

आ. २१

७. ज़मीन पर सीधे लेट जाईये । पैरों को जोड़कर रखें । दोनों बाज़ुओं को सिर के पीछे रखें । गहरी साँस लें, साँस को रोककर रखें । पैरों को ज़मीन से कुछ ईंच ऊपर ले जायें जबतक पेट के मध्य में अधिक तनाव महसूस नहीं होता (आ.२२) ।

दस गिनती करें । दस की गिनती तक रोकने के लिये कुछ अवधि लग सकती है । टाँगों को नीचे करें ।

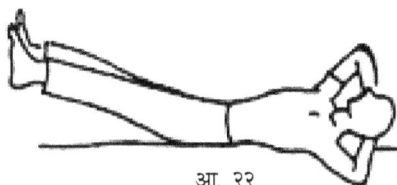

आ. २२

८. ऊपर बताये गये व्यायाम को टाँगों को फैलाये स्थिति में रखकर दोहरायें । इससे खिंचाव खासकर पेट के निचले और बाहरी हिस्से में महसूस होगा ।

९. पीठ के बल सीधे लेटें । बाज़ुओं को शरीर के साथ सीधे रखें । बायें कुल्हे और घुटने को मोड़कर बाज़ुओं से घुटने के नीचे पकड़ लें । घुटने को दायें कंधे की ओर ले जायें । दायें कंधे को भी आगे की ओर लायें । दाईं टाँग को सीधा रखें (आ. २३) । श्वास छोड़ने से मदद मिलती है । इसी व्यायाम को विपरीत टाँग से दोहरायें ।

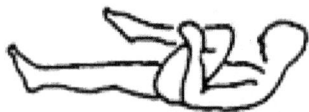
आ. २३

१०. सीधे लेट जायें । बाज़ुओं को सिर के पीछे सीधा तानकर रखें । उठकर हाथों की ऊँगलियों से पैरों की ऊँगलियों को छूने का प्रयास करें (आ. २४) ।

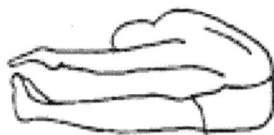
आ. २४

साँस छोड़ते हुए इसे करने से आसानी होगी । अगर शरीर के ऊपरी भाग को उठाने में कठिनाई हो तो किसी से टाँगों को नीचे दबाकर पकड़ने के लिये कहें , या पैरों की ऊँगलियों को किसी भारी फरनीचर , जैसे अलमारी , के नीचे फसा लें । अगर आप को पैरों की ऊँगलियों को छूने में कठिनाई हो रही हो तो टाँगों के जिस भाग तक ऊँगलियाँ पहुँच सकती हैं , उसे पकड़कर शरीर के ऊपरी भाग को नीचे खींचने का प्रयत्न करें और सिर को टाँगों के बीच रखने की कोशिश करें ।

ऊपर बताये गये सारे व्यायाम तीन–तीन बार करने चाहिये । इसे करने में लगभग सात मिनट का समय लगेगा । दिन में एक बार इसे करना पर्याप्त होगा किन्तु दर्द की स्थिति में दो बार की सलह दी जाती है ।

इस बात का ध्यान रखें कि रीढ़ की हड्डी को सामने की ओर झुकाने से मस्तिष्क से मेरूदंड निकलने वाली नली का घेरा बढ़ जाता है । इसके अलावा जिस छिद्र से मेरूदंड से निकली नस बाहर आती है , उसका घेरा भी बढ़ जाता है , जिससे नसों पर पड़ा दबाव कम हो जाता है । इसके अतिरिक्त और भी एक यह लाभ है कि इस तरह नीचे झुकने से शियाटिका से होने वाली वेदना कम हो जाती है ।

इस बात को समझना आवश्यक है कि कमर या पीठ के निचले भाग का दर्द और शियाटिका अन्य कई कारणों से भी हो सकता है । इसका समाधान, साधारण जाँच जैसे कि खून की जाँच और एक्स-रे द्वारा हो सकती है । ज़्यादातर पीठ के दर्द तनावपूर्ण हालातों की श्रेणी में आता है और पीठ के निचले भाग की देखभाल द्वारा इसका इलाज हो सकता है ।

अंत में , यह आवश्यक है कि हम मानसिक परेशानियों एवम तनावों से मुक्त होने का प्रयत्न करें , इसके लिये हमें तनावरहित रहने के तरीकों को सीखना होगा और जीवन जीने की कला को समझना होगा ।

दावा छूट:

इस किताब का विषय ज्यादातर यांत्रिक पीठ दर्दों के लिये है और संक्रमण, गांठ, वगैरह के लिये नहीं । पीठ के दर्द का कारण स्थापित करने के लिये, क्रिपया, डॉक्टर से सलह लें । इस किताब के विषयों का उपयोग करने से यदि कोई हानि पहुँचे (यद्यपि ऐसा कोई भी नहीं हुआ है), तो लेखक, अनुवादक, और प्रकाशक ज़िम्मेदार नहीं हैं ।

El dolor de la parte baja de la espalda y su cuidado

Dr. V. A. Mittal

MS (Orth.), MBBS, DPC

Cirujano Ortopeda

Traductora: Altagracia P. Mayers

Contenido

Entendiendo el dolor de la parte baja de la espalda y la ciática

El dolor de la parte baja de la espalda ocurre en el 80% al 97% de la población adulta, incapacitandola lo bastante hasta impedir la rutina normal, según reportaron diferentes personas que han trabajado en este tema. A nivel industrial, es la causa más común de horas de trabajo perdidas.

De acuerdo al desarrollo humano, la espina dorsal nunca fue concebida para soportar peso; su función era proteger la médula espinal. Sinembargo, la espina dorsal fue forzada a tomar esa función cuando el hombre evolucionó de cuadrúpedo a bípedo. Probablemente tomaría millones de años para que la espina dorsal se adaptara a su nueva función de soportar peso.

Hasta la edad de la adolescencia y aun desde temprano en la niñez, los huesos tienen una capa de cartílago, la cual siendo resistente, actúa como un amortiguador al compensar o disminuir el efecto de soportar peso, caminar, correr etc. Alrededor de la edad de 22 a 25 años, la mayor parte del cartílago se convierte en hueso relativamente más duro. La acción amortiguadora no ocurre efectivamente y hueso choca contra hueso, causando inflamación en las articulaciones (especialmente las que soportan peso), adherencias, sobrecrecimiento de las terminaciones etc; esto es la Osteoartrosis. El efecto acumulativo de esto se presenta como rigidez y dolor.

No se puede prevenir el envejecimiento pero, sus efectos se pueden prevenir cuidando la parte baja de la espalda; lo cual todo el mundo debe aprender al igual que el cuidado dental.

La espina dorsal si se mira del frente hacia atrás está supuesta a estar en una línea recta (fig. 1). Sinembargo, en mucha gente puede que esté curva. Las vértebras son los componentes esenciales de la espina dorsal o columna vertebral. En una espina curva, el espacio intervertebral se abre en el lado convexo y se acerca en el lado concavo como en una vara doblada. Esto causa presiones de diferentes niveles en las articulaciones vertebrales predisponiendolas a la osteoartrosis. Note que nervios provenientes de la médula espinal salen entre una vertebra y otra. Estos están en peligro de estar muy estirados o apretados, lo cual causa dolor que irradia desde la parte baja de la espalda hasta las extremidades inferiores, usualmente por la parte de atrás. A este dolor se le llama Ciática.

Cuando se mira la columna en forma lateral, esta tiene curvaturas naturales hacia adelante y hacia atrás como se muestra (fig. 2).

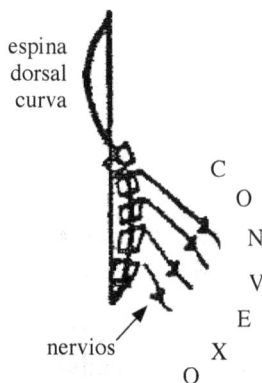

espina dorsal curva

CONVEX

nervios

Fig. 1

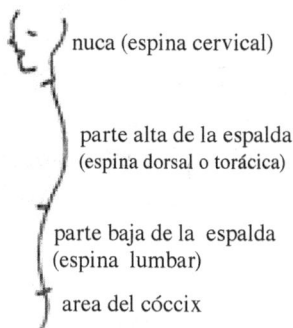

nuca (espina cervical)

parte alta de la espalda (espina dorsal o torácica)

parte baja de la espalda (espina lumbar)

area del cóccix

Fig. 2

La parte baja de la espalda curva hacia adelante y consiste en cinco vertebras (fig. 3). Cada vértebra presenta un par de procesos en la parte superior e inferior de cada lado de la línea media. Los procesos inferiores de la vértebra superior articulan con los respectivos procesos superiores de la vértebra inferior para formar articulaciones llamadas articulaciones facetarias. La articulación facetaria o sigoapositaria es una articulación lubricada y el frote constante de la superficie de la articulación la predispone a la inflamación.

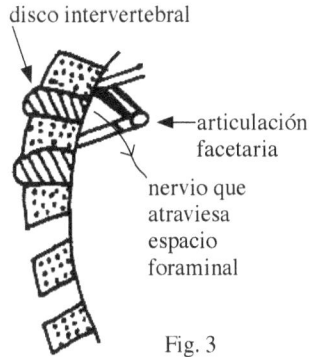

disco intervertebral

articulación facetaria

nervio que atraviesa espacio foraminal

Fig. 3

En el diagrama correspondiente es claro que si la articulación facetaria se vuelve artrítica o si sobresale el disco que está en medio de las vértebras, las raices nerviosas presentes en el orificio, como se muestra, pueden quedar afectadas provocando Ciática además de dolor en la parte baja de la espalda.

Mientras mas grande la profundidad de la curvatura hacia adelante, más grande es la posibilidad de inflamación en las articulaciones facetarias. Cuando tal inflamación (I) ocurre, produce dolor (D), lo cual produce espasmos (E) en los músculos de cada lado de la columna (la columna se siente como un canal longitudinal estrecho entre dos protuberancias longitudinales en cada lado formadas por los músculos) lo cual produce mas dolor (fig. 4).

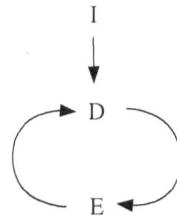

I
D
E

Fig. 4

De esta manera se establece un círculo vicioso que se puede manifestar como un dolor crónico y molestoso en la parte baja de la espalda con o sin exacerbaciones agudas e irradiación hacia las extremidades inferiores.

Qué aumenta la curvatura normal hacia adelante del área lumbar ? (fig. 5).

1. **Un incremento de la curvatura hacia atrás o sea una** corcoba en la parte superior de la espalda (mostrado por línea de puntos en la figura).

2. **Un abultamiento abdominal debido** a una debilidad de los músculos del abdomen, el embarazo o cargar peso en el frente como hacen las bibliotecarias, causaría una inclinación hacia adelante en la parte baja de la espalda.

diagrama

diagrama pélvico

vista lateral del hueso pélvico

inclinación

músculo del muslo

Fig. 5

3. **Músculos tensos en el muslo:** Estos músculos están unidos desde la parte de atrás de la pelvis hasta la parte de atrás de la rodilla. Si están tensos, causan una inclinación de la pelvis, a la cual está unida la columna y a consecuencia aumenta la inclinación hacia adelante.

4. **Zapatos de taco alto:** Es bien conocido que los zapatos de taco alto producen una postura especial. Esto es porque la pelvis esta inclinada hacia adelante desde arriba y lleva con ella la parte baja de la columna.

Muchas otras enfermedades (ex: infecciones) pueden tambien causar dolor en la parte baja de la espalda o causar Ciática (ex: Diabetes). Las mismas no se tratan en este artículo que se concentra en lo mecánico del dolor de la parte baja de la espalda. Tambien se sabe que situaciones que causan estrés mental y emocional causan dolor en la columna. Esto es debido a un estado de músculo tenso crónico y la traducción simbólica de llevar tales situaciones como una "carga" en la espalda.

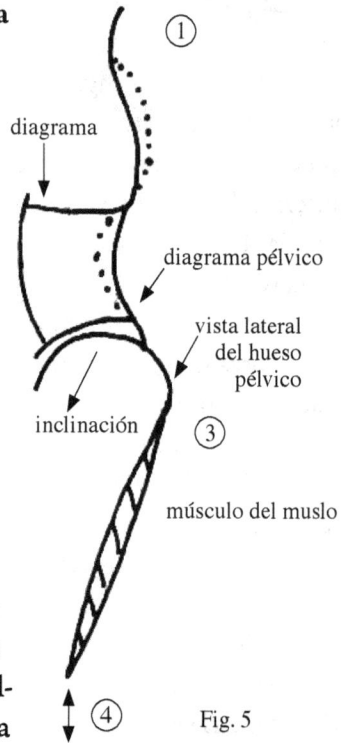

Cuidado de la parte baja de la espalda

Habiendo entendido el "por qué" del dolor de la parte baja de la espalda, el "cómo" del cuidado de la misma se vuelve fácil. Sinembargo, uno puede proceder a hacerlo aun no entendiendo la mecánica del dolor de la parte baja de la espalda.

Uno debe ser realista en cuanto a lo que espera. Ya que la prevención total del envejecimiento cronológico de la columna no es posible, uno solo puede retrasarlo y retrasar sus efectos. De manera que, relativamente, uno prevendría el dolor o disminuiría su amplitud y frecuencia (fig. 6).

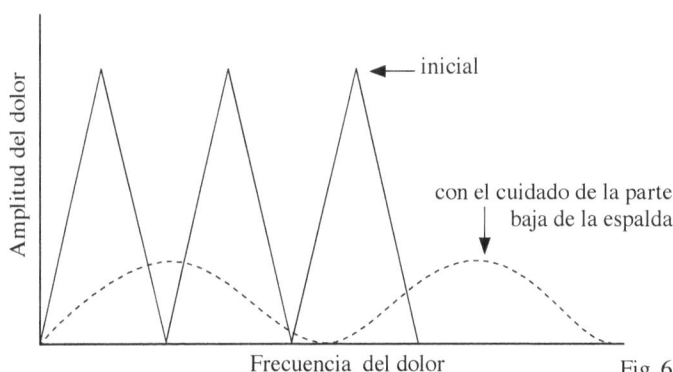

Fig. 6

Si el área lumbar de la columna está fuera de equilibrio, curva, tal como se ve desde el frente hacia atrás o viceversa, simplemente se corrige levantando el calzado en el lado convexo de la curva. Para encontrar desequilibrios por usted mismo, parese en frente a un espejo largo en ropa interior con los pies juntos, las extremidades superiores colgando. Hay un espacio natural entre los codos y la cintura. Esto es igual en una espina dorsal derecha pero, se disminuye en el lado convexo con aumento en el lado concavo en una espina dorsal curva. Para balancear esto, siga aumentando el calzado en un centímetro a la vez en el lado convexo (se puede usar planchas de madera o calzados con diferentes tamaños de tacos) hasta que el espacio se haga igual. Esto se puede confirmar pidiendole a otra persona u otro doctor que vea la espina dorsal desde atrás.

La desaparición completa del aumento de la curvatura hacia adelante del area lumbar de la columna se conseguiría fortaleciendo la musculatura abdominal, relajando los músculos de los muslos, estirando los músculos alrededor de la columna para aliviar los espasmos y dejar o reducir los tacones si se usan, especialmente durante episodios de dolor. Los de media pulgada a tres cuartos puede que esten bien. Si quiere lucir más alta es mejor usar plataforma.

Se necesita romper el círculo vicioso de inflamación, dolor y espasmos a través de mejorar la postura, hacer ejercicios, usar calor, medicamentos y cirugía (lo ultimo no se ha tratado aquí). La mayoria de los dolores de la parte baja de la espalda se pueden tratar con métodos conservadores.

Los medicamentos serían del grupo anti-inflamatorio primeramente, suplementados, si es necesario, con calmantes. Los medicamentos es mejor tomarlos con las comidas y con antiácidos para prevenir la irritación del tejido que cubre el estómago.

Calor, diatermia aplicada por un fisioterapista tambien se puede aplicar en la casa usando toallas humedas calientes. Cubra la espalda con la toalla y encima coloque un plástico para conservar el calor y la humedad. Cuando el dolor sea menos al tener los músculos relajados aproveche la oportunidad para practicar ejercicios. Note que las lámparas infra-rojas no proveen calor penetrante y como tal son inútiles.

Postura

Sentado(a): Uno no debe sentarse en la silla, tal como se nos ha enseñado, ocupando todo el asiento hasta pegar la espalda con el espaldar. Esto aumentaría la curvatura hacia adelante del área lumbar de la columna. Sientese más o menos en el frente del asiento con las rodillas levantadas, permitiendo que la parte baja de la espalda quede hacia adelante y la parte superior de la espalda pegada del respaldo del asiento. Uno podría cruzar el tobillo o la rodilla sobre la rodilla opuesta (fig. 7). Cuando esté sentado a la mesa, acerque la silla a la mesa y use el descanso para los pies que debe estar cerca del lado donde usted esta sentado (fig. 8). Si no hay un descanso, use una caja o gaveta para descansar sus pies. La idea es levantar las rodillas si es posible más altas que las caderas, de manera que incline la pelvis hacia adelante desde abajo y empujando la parte baja de la espalda hacia atrás. En la casa uno puede elegir sentarse en una superficie baja (fig. 9) de manera que las rodillas están automaticamente altas o siéntese sobre una superficie donde no le cuelguen los pies (fig 10).

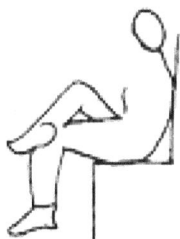

Fig. 7

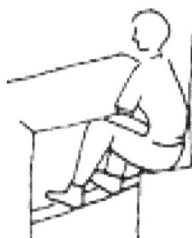

Fig. 8

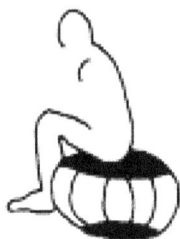

Fig. 9

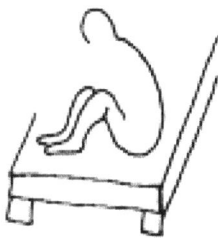

Fig. 10

Cuando esté en un vehículo, sinembargo, ocupe el asiento hasta el final y use una pequeña almohada para llenar el espacio entre la parte baja de la columna y el respaldo del asiento. Esto le va a ayudar a absorber los impactos verticales que reciba la espina dorsal. Si está manejando, además de lo que se ha dicho anteriormente, mantenga su asiento cómodamente cercano al freno y al acelerador de manera que las rodillas estén suficientemente elevadas.

Acostado(a): Use un colchón firme sobre una superficie de madera. Uno grueso y de algodón es el mejor. La espina dorsal se puede ahora ajustar sobre este. El piso duro es innecesario y lastima las protuberancias óseas.

Un colchón suave no permite que la columna se adapte sobre el. El acostarse boca abajo, sobre el estómago, se debe evitar ya que la parte baja de la espalda se mantiene doblada hacia atrás con una curva hacia adelante. Si se acuesta boca arriba, doble las rodillas, ponga los pies planos sobre la cama y use un almohadón o dos almohadas debajo de las rodillas para soporte. Esta postura aplana la parte lumbar de la columna sobre la cama (fig. 11). Si se acuesta de lado (sobre el izquierdo es más cómodo si se acuesta con un estómago lleno ya que recibe soporte). Las caderas y las rodillas deben de estar dobladas hacia el pecho. Una puede estar mas doblada que la otra (fig. 12)

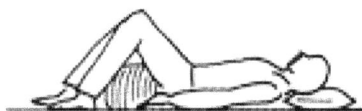

Fig. 11

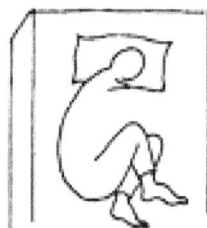

Fig. 12

De pie: Cuando sea posible, intermitentemente y concientemente, sientese o doblese hacia adelante y enderezese, esto quita mucho esfuerzo de la columna. Cuando uno esta parado derecho en ambos pies, la pelvis se mantiene en una posición trabada. Destrabando la pelvis intermitentemente a través de doblar ligeramente una rodilla y suavemente mover la pelvis hacia el lado opuesto, ayuda (fig. 13)

Trabajando en una posición de pie, como al cocinar, planchar etc, puede ser destructivo para la parte baja de la espalda. Lo que se debe y no se debe hacer se muestra en la figura 14. Mantenga la superficie de trabajo y su cuerpo cerca el uno del otro. Tener espacio para sus pies debajo de la superficie donde trabaja, ayuda. Use un banquito para sus pies pero vaya alternando un pies a la vez.

Caminando: De nuevo, intermitentemente sentarse o doblarse hacia delante, es muy bueno.

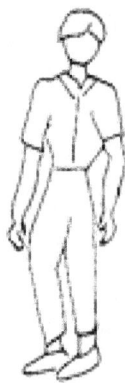

Fig. 13

Levantando peso: La espina dorsal está en su punto más débil cuando esta doblada hacia adelante. Imaginese los bloques con los

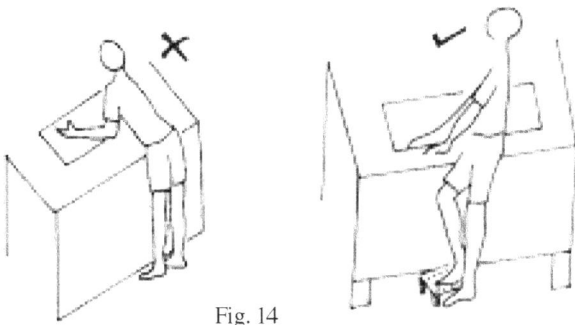

Fig. 14

que juegan los niños colocados verticalmente uno exactamente sobre otro. Un toque en la parte de arriba no los derriba. Sinembargo, si los colocara en una forma curva, se caerían fácilmente al tocarlos.

Cuando se carga peso en el frente con las extremidades inferiores más o menos rectas y la espina dorsal doblada hacia adelante, el fulcro (punto de apoyo) está en la columna y, al peso estar lejos, no hay ventaja mecánica, por lo tanto, se lastima la espalda. Cuando sea posible mantenga el peso cerca de usted pero a un lado. Doble las extremidades inferiores, mantenga la columna relativamente derecha y use los músculos de los muslos para ayudarse a levantar el peso al tiempo que endereza las extremidades inferiores (fig. 15)

Ejercicios

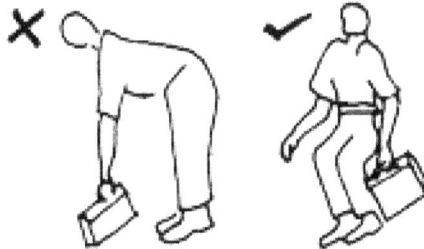

Fig. 15

Estos, junto con la buena postura, forman el pilar del cuidado de la parte baja de la espalda. El propósito de los ejercicios es estirar los músculos espasmódicos de alrededor de la columna, poner en forma la musculatura abdominal, relajar los músculos de los muslos, romper la adhesión en las coyunturas sinoviales y ayudar a la manipulación propia de la espina dorsal.

Ejercicios de pie

1. **Tocandose los dedos de los pies:** Con los pies casi juntos trate de tocarse los dedos de los pies al doblarse hacia adelante. No empiece a doblarse desde la cadera. Asegurese de doblar la espina dorsal mientras mantiene la cabeza cerca del cuerpo e ir doblando una vértebra trás otra (fig. 16). No es importante alcanzarse los dedos de los pies o el suelo sino doblarse lo más que pueda. Evite movimientos bruscos al irse doblando hacia adelante. Sinembargo, enderezarse de golpe es bueno. Exhalar mientras uno se va doblando, ayuda.

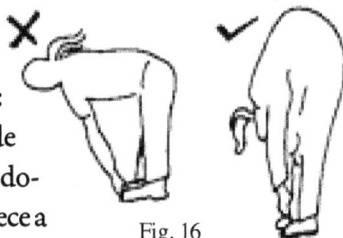

Fig. 16

2. **Giro y tirón:** Parese con los pies separados a una distancia de 1 a 1.5 pies, las manos en las caderas, doblese al máximo hacia la izquierda (fig. 17) Entonces ligeramente devuelva la rotación y gentilmente gire al máximo otra vez. Gire dos veces y entonces vuelva a la posicián neutral. Ahora doblese y repita la maniobra hacia la derecha. Si se tiene problemas en las rodillas, es mejor hacer este ejercicio sentado a la orilla de la cama o de una silla sin brazos. Esto va a evitar que se doble a la altura de las rodillas.

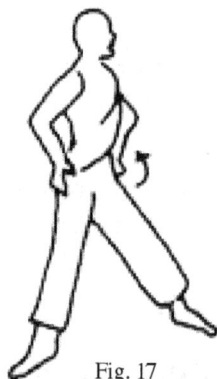

Fig. 17

3. **Toque cruzado:** Pies bien abiertos. Con los dedos de la mano derecha trate de cruzar y alcanzar los dedos del pie izquierdo (fig. 18). Vuelva a posición neutral. Repita con el lado contrario.

4. **Alterne dedos de los pies- calcañar-toque:** Pies bien separados. Con los dedos de la mano izquierda, intente tocar los dedos del pie izquierdo. Vuelva a posición neutral. Ahora trate de alcanzar con los dedos de la mano derecha el calcañar derecho (fig. 19). Vuelva a neutral. Hagalo con el lado contrario.

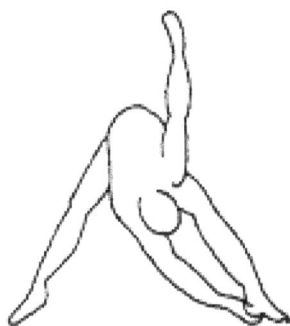

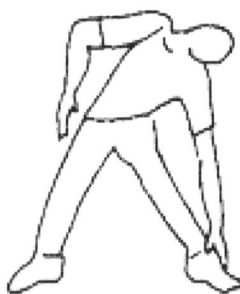

Fig. 18   Fig. 19

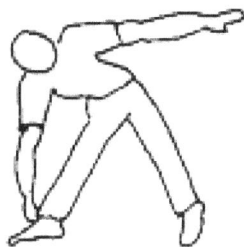

5. Doblandose de lado: Los pies bien separados. Las extremidades superiores estiradas a cada lado del cuerpo. Doblese hacia la izquierda, colocando el brazo izquierdo a lo largo de la pierna izquierda. Estire el brazo derecho hacia arriba y dirija su mirada hacia allí (fig. 20). Vuelva a posición neutral. Repita los movimientos con el lado derecho.

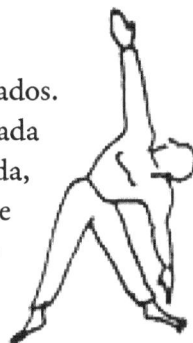

Fig. 20

6. Pateando: Tome uno o dos pasos hacia adelante y levante la pierna izquierda hasta tocar los dedos de la mano izquierda que debe estar hasta la altura del hombro (fig. 21). Cuidese de no resbalarse y caerse (fig. 20) hacia atrás. Evite suelos o calzados resbalozos. Repita con el lado derecho.

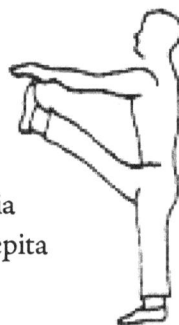

Ejercicios de suelo

Fig. 21

(por ejemplo sobre una superficie dura y firme tienda una manta de suelo)

7. Las manos detrás de la cabeza. Los pies juntos. Estire las extremidades inferiores. Inhale, no deje salir el aire. Levante los pies unas cuantas pulgadas hasta que sienta el máximo esfuerzo a la mitad del abdomen. Aguante hasta que cuente hasta diez (esto pueda que requiera ir poco a poco hasta que pueda llegar hasta diez con el tiempo). Luego bajelos (fig. 22).

---

8. Repita lo anterior con los pies bien abiertos. El esfuerzo se siente mayormente en la parte baja y exterior del abdomen.

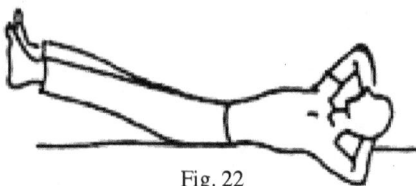

Fig. 22

9. Acuestese boca arriba, los brazos a los lados. Doble la cadera y la rodilla izquierda y agarrese la pierna justamente debajo de la rodilla con las dos manos. Llevese la rodilla hacia el hombro derecho el cual puede estar arqueado hacia adelante. Mantenga la otra pierna derecha (fig. 23). Exhalar ayuda. Repita con los lados opuestos.

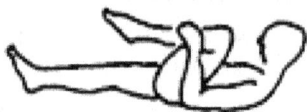

Fig. 23

10. Acuestese boca arriba, los brazos hacia arriba y detrás de la cabeza. Levantese y trate de alcanzarse los dedos de los pies (fig. 24). Exhalar ayuda. Si usted no puede levantarse, pidale a alguien que le sostenga las piernas o meta los dedos de los pies debajo de un mueble pesado, tal vez una alacena, para que se ayude. Si no puede alcanzarse los dedos de los pies, agarrese cualquier parte de la pierna que alcance y halese hacia delante como si intentara enterrar la cabeza entre las piernas.

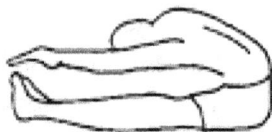

Fig. 24

Todos los ejercicios anteriores son para hacerse tres veces cada uno. Toma unos 7 minutos. Una vez al dia es usualmente suficiente. Es recomendable hacerlos dos veces al dia si tiene dolor.

Se sabe que el doblar la espina dorsal hacia adelante aumenta el espacio del canal en la columna vertebral a través del cual la médula espinal desciende desde el cerebro. Tambien aumenta el espacio foraminal quitando asi presión de los nervios. Esto es un beneficio adicional en cuanto a dolor neural que se irradia.

Precaución: Muchas otras condiciones pueden producir dolor en la parte baja de la espalda y Ciática. Estas se pueden descartar a través de la investigacion simple, frecuentemente examenes de sangre y rayos-x. Sinembargo, la mayoria de los dolores de espalda caen en la categoria del fenómeno de músculos muy esforzados o muy trabajados y se pueden atender con tratamiento para la parte baja de la espalda.

Finalmente, los estreses sicológicos se deben atender mediante el aprendizaje de tecnicas de relajamiento y el entender el arte de vivir.

Excepción de responsabilidad

La información en este libro esta dirigida mayormente hacia la mecánica del dolor de la parte baja de la espalda y no para infecciones, tumores, etc. Por favor consulte a su médico para establecer la causa del dolor de la parte baja de su espalda. El autor, los traductores y la casa editorial no se hacen responsables de cualquier daño que pudiera resultar por utilizar el contenido de este libro (aunque no se sabe de ninguno que haya ocurrido).

Doulè nan Senti ak Swen Pou Senti

Dr. V. A. Mittal

MS (Orth.), MBBS, DPC

Chirijyen Òtopedis

Tradiksyon : Idi Jawarakim

Tabdèmatyè (apèsu)

Ann konprann doulè nan senti ak sayatika

Doulè nan senti afekte ant 80 a 97% (pousan) nan popilasyon adilt-la nan yon pwen ke anpil diferan travayè rapòte ke yo pa ka fè aktivite regilye-yo lè yo santi-l. Se rezon ki fè pifò moun pa al travay lè yo malad.

Zo rèl do-a okòmansman pat vrèman fèt pou sipòte pwa kò-nou. Sèl fonksyon-li se te pou pwoteje pati nan sèvo-a ki fè yon branch rive jouk nan zo kroupyon-an. Lè imen-an vin aprann mache, de 4 pat a 2 pye, zo rèl do-a vin fòse ranpli fonksyon pote pwa kò-a tou. Sa ka petèt pran kèk milyon ane anvan zo rèl do-a vin adapte a nouvo wòl pote pwa anlè kò-nou.

Jouk nou rive nan laj pou n'fòme oubyen menm lè nou nan kòmansman ventèn-nou-yo konsa, zo nou-yo kouvri ak yon kouch zo krip trè rezistan, ki fòme yon kousen ki absòbe pwa kò-a, sekous mache, sekous kouri, elatriye. Letan nou gen 22 a 25 an-yo konsa, pifò nan zo krip sa-yo transfòme e yo vin di. Kousen-an vin pa la ankò, e zo vin ap frote yonn kont lòt ki vin lakòz zo jwenti-yo ap anfle sitou jwenti ki sipòte pwa kò nou (tankou jenou-yo konsa). Sa konn lakòz tou dèfwa yon kondisyon ki rele adezyon kote 2 zo ki fwote ansanm vin ap kole sou deyò, osnon pwent zo-yo vin ap grandi twò long eksetera, ki vin bay rimatis nan zo. Lè nou adisyone tout bagay sa-yo, k'ap rive tout tan, zo-yo vin rèd e nou gen doulè.

Nou pa ka anpeche-n laj rantre sou nou, men nou ka redui efè laj fè sou tay-nou si nou pran swen senti-nou—yon bagay tout moun ta sipoze aprann menm jan nou aprann pran swen dan-nou. Sepandan, li ta yon bònide si nou te aprann kijan doulè nan senti fonksyone anvan nou kòmanse bay senti-a swen.

Si yon moun ap gade chini do-nou devan rive sou dèyè, li ta sipoze wè yon liy dwat (desen 1). Men se konsa tou, zo rèl do anpil moun ka on jan koube. Zo-yo ki fòme kolòn vètèbral-la rele vètèb. Nan yon kolòn vètebral ki koube, espas-yo ki nan mitan vèteb-yo louvri plis sou kote ki bonbe-a, e yo pi fèmen sou kote ki fè basen-an tankou yon ti branch bwa ki pliye. Sa vin kreye plis presyon sou yon bò nan kolòn vètebral-la, ki fè li vin pi fasil pou yon moun fè rimatis nan zo. Obsève byen, ke se nan espas ki nan mitan vètèb kolòn vètebral-yo, nè-yo sòti. Nè sa-yo ka menase—yo ka swa twò detire, swa twò kwense. Sa vin kreye yon doulè ki sòti depi nan senti desann tout dèyè janm ou. Doulè sa-a rele syatik (sayatika an angle).

Lè n'ap gad yon moun de pwofil kolòn vètèbral-li fè koub e al devan, e al dèyè (desen 2).

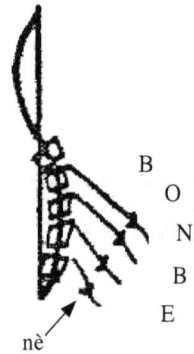

yon kolòn vertebral ki kwochi

B
O
N
B
E

nè

Desen 1

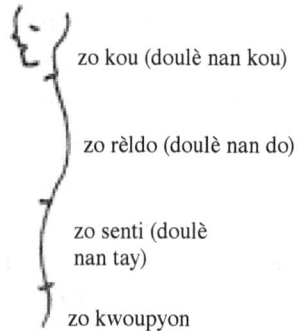

zo kou (doulè nan kou)

zo rèldo (doulè nan do)

zo senti (doulè nan tay)

zo kwoupyon

Desen 2

Koub senti-a al devan, epi li gen 5 vètèb (desen 3). Chak vètèb-yo boujonnen 2 chouk, e anwo e anba, sou chak bò zo rèl do-a—liy nan mitan-an. Boujon anba yon vètèb rankontre ak boujon anlè vètèb ki anba li-a pou yo fòme nouvo jwenti yo rele "facet joints" an angle. Facet joint-la se yon jwenti ki librifye; e lè l'ap fwote tout tan, sa vin rann-li pi fasil pou li anfle.

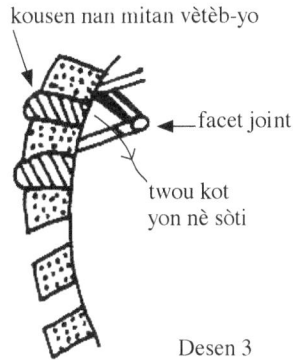

kousen nan mitan vètèb-yo

facet joint

twou kot yon nè sòti

Desen 3

Selon desen-an, li klè ke si facet joint-yo vin devlope rimatis oubyen si yon disk (yon ti kousen won kon plimo) ta vin kòmkwadire kwense tankou yon sandwitch nan mitan 2 vètèb, kòm nou ka wè-l nan desen-an, rasin nè-a k'ap sòti nan twou-a (foramen) ka vin menase, epi li ka vin lakòz syatik/sayatika anplis doulè nan senti.

Plis koub sou devan-an pi pwononse, se pi plis chans ki genyen tou pou facet joints-yo anfle. Lè anflamasyon (A) sa-yo rive, yo bay gwo doulè (D) ki vin lakòz misk (M)-yo (vyann kò-a) ki toude bò zo rèl do-a ap danse. Zo rèl do-a fè tankou yon fant ki desann sòti anwo ki nan mitan 2 bit misk ki vin lakoz plis doulè (desen 4). Se nan konsa yon sèk visye (kote gen 2 bagay, yonn ap lakòz lòt san rete) ki ka swa vin prezante yon doulè senti malouk ki la touttan, li ka byen agrave doulè-a epi fè-l deplase desann nan janm-yo, konsa tou, li ka pa fè anyen ditou.

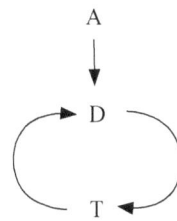

A

D

T

Desen 4

Kisa ki ka fè koub nòmal zo do-a, nan nivo senti-nou vin pi pwononse? (desen 5)

1. **Koub anlè do-a vin pi pwononse,** yon bòs nan anlè do-a (liy tipwen tipwen ki nan desen-an)

2. Misk nan vant-yo vin febli, ki vin lakòz **vant-la vide**, gwosès, pote chay devan tankou moun ki pran abitid pote liv devan-yo, tout bagay sa-yo ka vin lakòz bafon nan senti-a vin pi pwononse.

3. Lè **misk dèyè janm-yo vin ap redi**, misk sa-yo tache sòti nan zo basen-an sou dèyè, rive jouk nan dèyè zo jenou-yo. Si misk sa-yo rèd, yo lakòz zo basen-yo, ki tache ak zo rèl do-a, redi vin sou devan; sa fòse koub zo rèl do-a, nan nivo tay-la, vin pi pwononse.

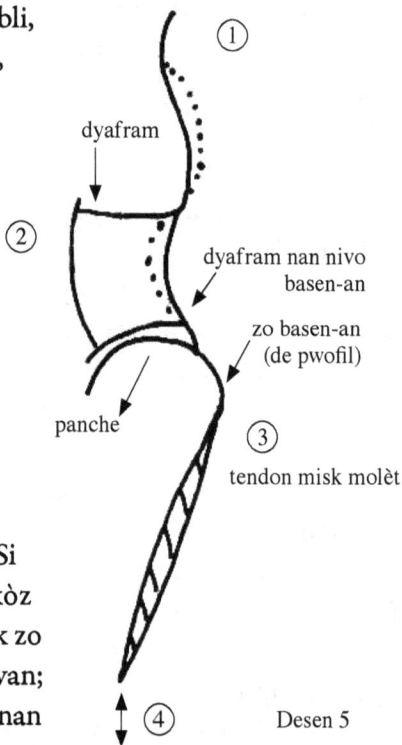

dyafram

① dyafram

② dyafram nan nivo basen-an

zo basen-an (de pwofil)

panche

③ tendon misk molèt

④ Desen 5

4. **Talon kikit:** Tout moun konnen ke talon kikit fòse yon moun mache bwòdè. Rezon-an se basen-an ki vin panche vin sou devan depi sou anwo e sa fòse zo rèl do-a pliye vin sou devan tou.

Gen anpil lòt kondisyon tou ki ka lakòz doulè nan senti (pa egzanp enfeksyon), osnon syatik/sayatika (pa egzanp dyabèt). Nou pap vrèman diskite kondisyon sa-yo andetay nan ti liv-sa ki plis konsantre sou mekanism doulè nan senti-a. Nou konnen ke sekous tèt chaje, estrès mantal ak emosyonèl ka lakòz nou gen doulè nan senti-n tou. Rezon-an se misk nan do-w yo vin nan yon eta kote ke yo toujou redi; kòmkwadire yon moun ki toujou ap pote yon chay sou do-l. Kidonk, se sa ki fè nou di ke moun sa-a ap pote yon chay "envizib" sou do-l.

Swen Pou Tay-Nou

Infwa yon moun fin konprann kisa ki lakòz doulè nan senti, sa vin rann li pi fasil pou nou pran swen do-li. Menm lè yon moun pa konn mekanism doulè nan senti, li toujou kapab suiv konsèy sa-yo. Fòk nou reyalis tou antèm de kisa n'ka atann-nou kòm rezilta. Nou pa ka totalman anpeche laj afekte zo rèl do-nou. Plis nou ka fè, se retade limenm ak tout bagay ki vin avè-l yo. Pou rezon sa-a, yon moun ka rezonableman evite doulè, ou menm redui fòs-li ou menm diminye ki kantite fwa li santi doulè-a (desen 6).

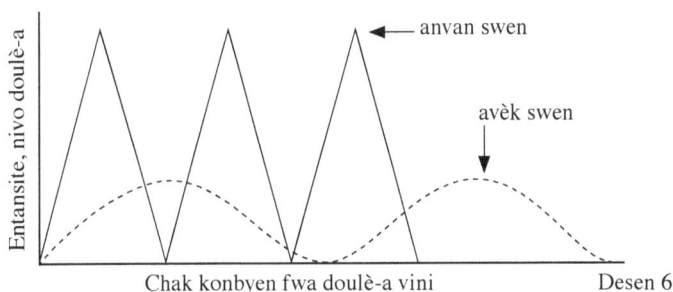

Desen 6

Si zo rèl do-a, nan nivo senti-a, pa byen balanse, si li kwochi lè nou gade on moun anfas oubyen pa do, nou ka korije pwoblèm-nan si nou annik fè semèl soulye ki sou bò ki bonbe-a vin ontijan piwo. Si ou vle tcheke pou ou wè si pwòp zo rèl do pa-w kwochi, kanpe devan yon glas kote ou ka wè tout kò-w, an kalson osnon an kilòt sèlman. Pandye 2 bra-w.

Gen yon espas natirèl ant koud bra-w ak flan-ou. Si zo rèl do-w dwat, espas-la sipoze menm gwosè-a nan toulède bò-yo. Si zo rèl do-w pa dwat, espas-la sipoze pi piti sou bò ki bonbe-a, e li pi gwo sou bò ki fè fon-an. Pou fè toulède bò-yo vin menm gwosè, mete yon ti mòso planch 1 santimèt epesè anba semèl soulye ki sou bò ki bonbe-a. Ajoute 1 santimèt anplis alafwa (ou ka eseye met 2 soulye ki gen talon-yo diferan otè) jiskaske espas ant flan-ou ak 2 koud bra-yo vin menm nan toulède bò. Ou ka fè yon lòt moun osnon yon doktè verifye zo rèl do-a tou.

Pou elimine gwo koub kolòn vètebral-la fè vin sou devan-an, nan nivo senti-a, sa ap mande non sèlman ke misk ki nan vant-yo vin pi djanm, ansuit fè misk nan molèt-yo vin pi lache, epitou ap gen bezwen pou detire misk ki fè tout longè zo rèl do-a tou; pou yo pa ap tresayi. Yon lòt bagay k'ap bezwen fèt tou, se evite met talon wo osnon redui otè talon on moun mete, de demi a twaka pous, sitou nan moman kote li gen doulè. Si yon moun ta vle parèt piwo, li ta preferab ke li mete yon soulye a semèl pwès.

Laviwonn ant anflamasyon, doulè, ak tresayman misk kote yonn ap lakòz lòt-la san rete, sipoze korije avèk fason ou pote kò-w, fè egzèsis, chalè, medikaman, ak fè operasyon (nou pap diskite aspè sa-a). Pifò doulè nan tay ka soulaje avèk dè mwayen ki pa twò drastik.

Medikaman prensipal-yo ta sipoze konbat anflamasyon, e si li nesesè, ak doulè tou. Li ta miyò si nou pran medikaman sa-yo ak manje e antiasid pou anpeche-yo irite lestomak-ou.

Apade tretman "diathermy" (kote yon teknisyen sèvi ak yon espès de kouran elektrik pou li chofe yon tisi osnon yon gwoup tisi) ke yon fizyoterapis fè nan yon klinik, yon moun ka met konprès dlo cho sou do-li. Konprès-la ta sipoze kouvri ak yon plastik pou li ka konsève chalè ak tout imidite. Lè misk-yo fin lache ase pou doulè-a bese, pwofite; se yon bon lè pou fè egzèsis. Note ke lanp enfrawouj-yo pa bay chalè ki penetre fon; kidonk, yo pa vrèman fè ankenn efè.

Fason yon moun pote kò-li

Chita: Yon moun pa ta sipoze chita jouk dèyè nan yon chèz tankou yo te toujou aprann-nou pou nou chita. Pozisyon sa-a ka fè zo senti-a koube twòp vin sou devan. Chita sou devan chèz-la ak jenou-yo soulve nan yon fason pou ou ka pèmèt zo ren-an al pi devan. Nou te ka kwaze swa yon jepye sou yon jenou, swa yon jenou sou lòt jenou-an (desen 7). Lè ou chita atab, rale chèz-la vin pi pre tab-la epi sèvi ak bawo tab-la ki ta sipoze pre-ou bò tab-la (desen 8). Si tab-la pa gen bawo, sèvi ak yon bwat osnon yon tiwa pou repoze pye-w yo. Ide-a se fè jenou-yo vin pi wo ke zo kwis-yo si li posib, yon fason pou tablati basen-an panche vin sou devan; apati de anba-w ki pouse zo senti-w al dèyè. Lò-w lakay-ou ou ka chita sou yon bagay ki ba (desen 9) defason ke jenou-yo vin otomatikman piwo; osnon, ou ka met pye-w sou kèlkeswa bagay ou chita-a (desen 10). Men lè yon moun nan yon machin, li ta sipoze chita jouk nan fon kousen-an nèt, epi sèvi ak yon ti zòrye pou fin ranpli espas ant do kousen-an e senti-l. Sa te ka ede absòbe chòk ou te ka resevwa lè ou nan yon machin sou yon wout kraze. Si yon moun ap kondui, li ta bon tou si li avanse kousen chofè-a pre pedal-yo yon fason pou jenou-yo ka wo ase.

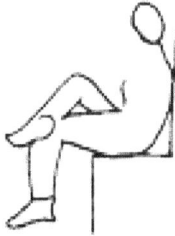
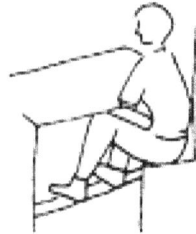

Desen 7   Desen 8

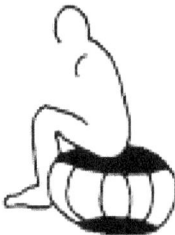
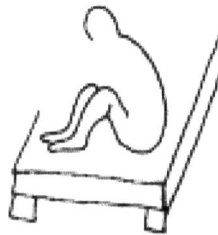

Desen 9   Desen 10

Kouche: Sèvi ak yon matla ki di sou yon planche. Yon matla koton ki pwès pi bon toujou; zo rèl do-a ka ajiste-l a li. Kouche atè nan yon planche pa nesesè; sa te ka fè pwent zo-yo mal tou.

Yon matla ki mou pa vrèman pèmèt zo rèl do-a adapte-l toutbon vre. Evite kouche sou vant puiske zo senti-a ki natirèl-man pliye al dèyè vin fè yon koub vin sou devan. Si ou kouche apla sou do, pliye jenou-yo, mete pye-yo apla sou matla-a; sèvi ak yon kousen long osnon 2 zòrye anba dèyè jenou-yo kòm sipò. Pozisyon sa-a vin fè zo senti-nou vin apla sou matla-a (desen 11).

(Si nou kouche sou kan, l'ap pi alèz pou ou kouche sou bò goch sitou si vant-ou plen; sa sipòte lestomak-la). Pliye zo kuis-yo ak zo jenou-yo kòmkwa ou ta vle fè yon jenou touche kòf lestomak-ou. Yon jenou ka piwo ke lòt-la (desen 12).

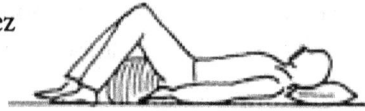

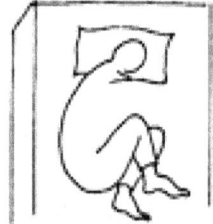

Desen 11

Si yon moun pran abitid, lè li posib, pou li chita pliye kò-l al sou devan, epi drese kò-l vit, sa te ka soulaje zo rèl do-a anpil. Lè li kanpe dwat sou toulède janm-yo, zo tablati basen-an rete bloke nan yon sèl pozisyon. Si detanzantan, li pliye yon jenou, epi fè menm bagay-la ak lòt-la defason ke hanch-li-yo woule debò, pa twò fò, sa bay yon soulajman tou (desen 13).

Desen 12

Yon moun ki travay kanpe, tankou fè manje, osnon pase rad elatriye, sa te ka vrèman deranje zo senti-a. Nan (desen 14)-la, nou montre kisa yon moun ka fè, ak kisa li pa dwe fè. Li dwe kanpe pre ak bagay kote li ap travay-la. Si li kite espas pou pye-l anba kote l'ap travay-la, sa te ka ede tou. Mete yon ti tabourè/bankèt anba yon pye, epi chanje pye detanzantan.

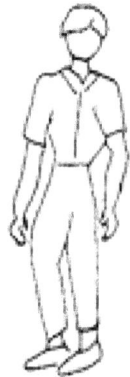

Mache: Yon lòt fwa ankò, lè yon moun ap mache, li bon pou l'ta fè yon chita detanzantan, oubyen pou li pliye kò-l al devan, epi apre, drese kò-l rapid.

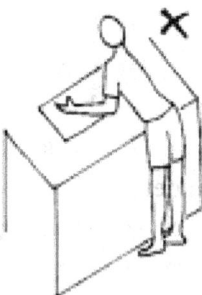

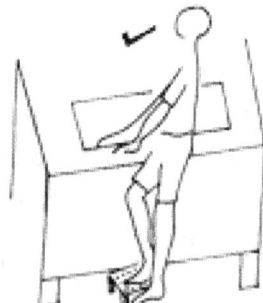

Desen 13

Desen 14

Leve Chay: Zo rèl do-n pi frajil lè li pliye al sou devan. Fè vizyon blòk anbwa timoun konn ap jwe avè-yo-a. Si nou fè yon pil ak blòk sa-yo, yonn sou lòt, kanpe dwat, epi nou frappe sa ki anlè nèt-la, se pa yo tout k'ap tonbe. Men tou, si pil-la on jan kwochi, tout blòk-yo ka tonbe fasil lè nou frappe-yo. Lè nou pote chay sou devan, ak janm-nou plizoumwen dwat, epi zo rèl do-nou plizoumwen pliye al sou devan, se zo rèl do-a ki bay tout sipò-a, e chay-la ki pa pre kò nou, vin yon dezavantaj mekanik (chay-la nan yon move pozisyon) ki lakòz zo rèl do-a fè twòp efò. Nenpòt lè li posib, pote yon chay sou kote kò-nou epi pre kò-nou tou. Pliye jwenti nan janm-nou, kuis-nou osnon jenou-nou, kenbe kolòn vètebral-la pi dwat ke nou kapab, epi sèvi ak misk kuis-nou pou ede-n leve chay-la lè nou drese janm-nou (desen 15).

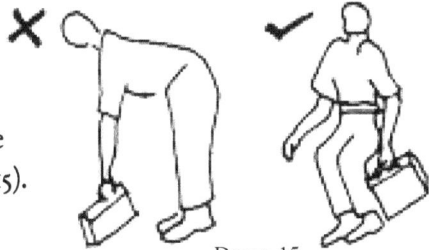

Egzèsis

Desen 15

Fè egzèsis ansanm avèk fason osnon pozisyon nou pòte kò-nou, se meyè bagay nou te ka fè pou nou kenbe senti-nou ansante. Egzèsis sa-yo fèt pou detire misk ki tout longè rèl do-a, ki dèfwa konn ap redi, fè misk nan vant-nou-yo vin pi solid, lache misk mòlèt-nou-yo, detache 2 zo jwenti ki pa ta sipoze kole (jwenti synovial) epi pèmèt zo rèl do-a tou bouje poukont-li.

Egzèsis pandan ou kanpe:

1. **Touche zòtèy-ou:** Kole 2 pye-w ansanm. Eseye pliye devan jouk nou touche zòtèy-yo. Kenbe janm-yo

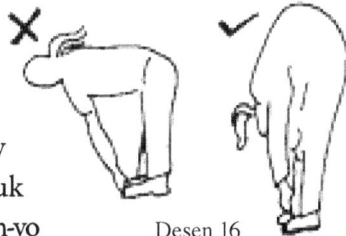

Desen 16

dwat depi nan hanch-ou epi glise desann... Fè de fason pou tèt-ou pre kò-w (touche anba kou-w ak manton-w) epi pliye zo rèl do-a yon ne alafwa (desen 16). Sa ki pi enpòtan-an se pa tèlman touche zòtèy-ou osnon atè-a, men se repete menm mouvman-an otan ou kapab. Evite bay kò-w gwo sekous lè w'ap desann. Drese kò-w rapid bon pou ou. Lage souf-ou lè w'ap glise desann.

2. **Tòdye ak sekous:** Ekate pye-w yonn a yon pye edmi konsa, epi met 2 men-w nan hanch-ou. Tòdye hanch-ou agoch otan ke ou kapab (desen 17). Detòdye hanch-ou dousman epi yon grenn kou, retounen-l ak yon ti sakad, nan menm pozisyon-an agoch ankò. Repete mouvman sa-a 2 fwa epi retounen nan pozisyon nòmal-ou, sètadi dwat devan-w. Konnyè-a, fè menm mannèv ou te fè sou bò goch-la sou bò dwat-la. Si ou gen pwoblèm nan jenou, li t'ap miyò pandan w'ap fè egzèsis sa-a, si ou te chita jouk devan sou yon chèz ki pa gen manch, osnon sou yon kabann. Konsa, sa va anpeche ou fè jefò (tòdye) sou jenou-w.

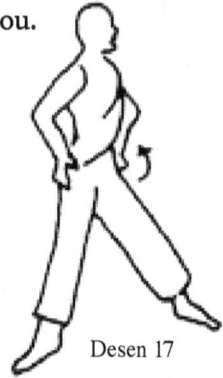

Desen 17

3. **Touche zòtèy antravè:** Ekate pye-w byen gran. Pliye senti-w epi eseye touche zòtèy pye goch-ou ak dwèt men dwat-ou (desen 18). Retounen nan pozisyon ou te kòmanse-a, epi refè menm mannèv-la sou lòt bò-a.

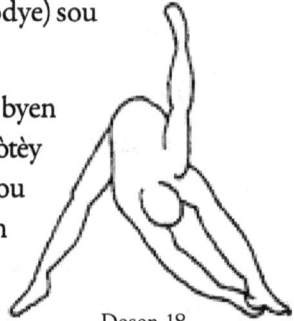

Desen 18

4. **Touche zòtèy epi talon sou menm bò-a:** Ekate pye-w byen gran. Ak dwèt men goch-ou, eseye touche zòtèy pye goch-ou, eseye touche zòtèy-yo ki sou menm bò-a. Retounen nan pozisyon ou te kòmanse-a. Konnyè-a, fè menm bagay-la ak men e zòtèy pye dwat-ou (desen 19).

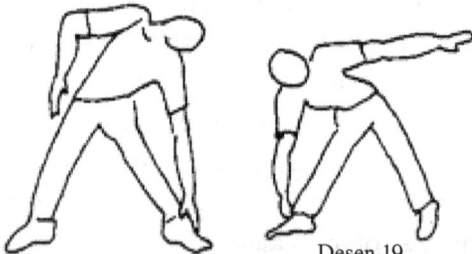

Desen 19

Low Back Pain and Low Back Care

5. **Pliye sou kote:** Ekate 2 pye-w, lonje 2 bra-w sou kote-w. Pliye sou kote goch-ou. Pou men goch-la ka glise sou janm goch-ou. Leve bra dwat-la anlè epi gade nan direksyon-l (desen 20). Retounen nan pozisyon ou te komanse-a epi refè menm mannèv-la sou lòt bò-a.

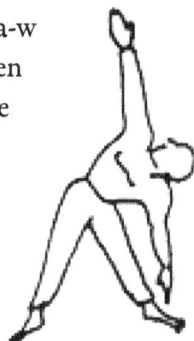

Desen 20

6. **Tire pye-w anlè:** Leve bra goch-ou toudwat devan-w rive otè zepòl-ou konsa (desen 21). Fè yonn ou 2 pa annavan epi lanse pye goch-ou anlè jouk pou ou arive touche dwèt men goch-ou. Fè atansyon pou ou pa tonbe al sou dèyè; evite fè egzèsis sa-yo si atè kote ou kanpe-a glise, si ou kanpe sou anyen ki glise. Evite mete soulye ki glise tou. Lè ou fin fè egzèsis sa-a sou yon bò, fè-li sou lòt bò-a tou.

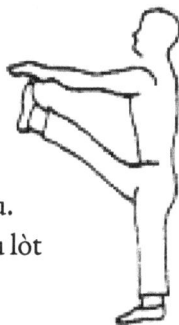

Desen 21

Egzèsis pandan ou kouche
(sou yon bagay ki di, pa egzanp, yon lenn ou mete atè)

7. Met men-w dèyè tèt-ou, kole 2 pye-w. Detire toulède janm-ou-yo toudwat. Rale yon souf, kenbe-l. Soulve 2 janm-yo kèlke pous de atè-a jouk ou kòmanse santi misk nan mitan vant-ou-yo kòmanse redi. Konte jiska 10 pandan ou nan pozisyon sa-a (desen 22—sa ka pran-w kèlke tan anvan ou ka arive kenbe pozisyon sa-a jouk ou arive konte jiska 10). Lè ou fini, bese janm-yo.

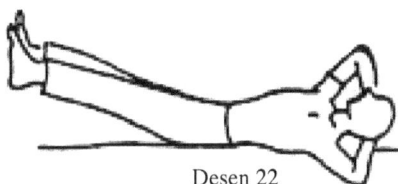

Desen 22

8. Repete menm egzèsis-la. Sètfwasi ekate janm-yo. Ou gen pou santi redi-a plis nan flan-yo ak anbativant-ou.

9. Kouche apla sou do ak 2 bra-yo sou kote-w. Pliye kuis ak je-nou goch-la epi kwaze dwèt-yo imedyatman anba jenou-an pou sipòte-l. Pliye jenou-an nan direksyon zepòl dwat-ou ke ou koube yontikras vin devan. Kenbe janm dwat-la apla tou dwat (desen 23). Lage souf-ou rann egzèsis-la pi fasil. Fè menm egzèsis-la sou lòt bò-yo.

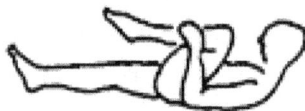

Desen 23

10. Kouche apla, detire ponyèt-ou piwo epi dèyè tèt-ou. Drese kò-w epi eseye touche zòtèy-yo (desen 24). Lage souf-ou ka ede-w. Si ou drese kò-w, mande yon moun pou met presyon sou 2 janm-ou-yo, osnon foure zòtèy-ou-yo anba yon mèb ki lou te ka ede-w tou. Si ou pa ka touche zòtèy-yo kenbe kèlkeswa pati nan janm-nan ou kapab kenbe, epi rale kò-w desann kòmkwa ou t'ap eseye foure tèt-ou nan mitan janm-ou.

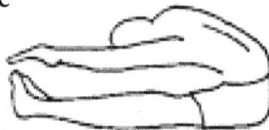

Desen 24

Ou ta sipoze fè chak egzèsis sa-yo 3 fwa. Sa ka pran antou 7 minit. Yon fwa pa jou ta sipoze kont. Si ou gen doulè, fè-yo 2 fwa.

Note ke pliye al sou devan gen avantaj agrandi espas nan kanal anndan vètèb-la, kote pati nan sèvo-a ki desann al jouk nan zo kroupyon-an, pase. Li vin fè twou nan espas kote nè-yo pase vin pi gran tou. Se yon avantaj anplis nan ka kote ou gen nè k'ap ba-w doulè.

Yon dènye mo atansyon. Gen anpil lòt kondisyon ki ka lakòz doulè nan senti osnon sayatika. Nou ka al pifon nan kesyon-an jeneralman si nou annik fè egzamen san, osnon radyografi pou nou elimine posiblite ke doulè sa-yo te ka gen yon lòt kòz. Sepandan, pifò doulè nan tay rantre nan kategori fo mouvman e yo ka trete si nou suiv konsè nou li nan liv sa-a.

Finalman, ou ka elimine estrès tèt chaje si ou senpman aprann teknik pou ou rilaks-ou ak konpran kijan ou ta vrèman sipoze viv lavi-a.

Yon mo atansyon:

Enfòmasyon nan liv sa-a ap sèvi pou pifò doulè nan senti. Nou pa konseye-l pou enfeksyon, timè, elatriye. Tanpri, wè ak yon doktè ki va di kisa ki lakòz doulè senti-a. Moun ki ekri liv-la, tradiktè-yo, ak moun ki pibliye liv-la, pa responsab pou ankenn domaj (kwak sa pa janm rive) ki te ka rive pandan ou ap sèvi ak enfòmasyon nan liv-la.

Dor Lombar e Cuidados com a Coluna Lombar

Dr. V. A. Mittal
MS (Orth.), MBBS, DPC
Cirurgião Ortpédico

Tradutora: Patricia B.P. Dos Santos

Conteúdo

Compreendendo a dor lombar e a dor ciática

A dor nas costas ocorre em 80% a 97% da população adulta incapacitando a pessoa a ponto de impedí-la de sua rotina normal como relatada por vários pesquisadores no assunto. É a causa mais comum de perda de mão-de-obra no trabalho.

A espinha foi desenvolvida somente para proteger a medula espinhal e não para carregar peso. No entanto, a espinha foi obrigada à assumir essa função quando o ser humano evoluiu de quadrúpede para bípede. Provavelmente, levaria milhões de anos para que a coluna se adaptasse à sua nova função de carregar peso.

Até a adolescência e mesmo no príncipio da vida adulta, os ossos possuem uma camada de cartilagem que, sendo maleável, age como um amortecedor que absorve o choque de carregar o peso, caminhar, correr, etc. Ao atingir os 22 aos 25 anos de idade, a maioria dessa cartilagem já foi absorvida por ossos que tornaram-se relativamente duros. Nessa altura, a amortização não ocorre tão efetivamente e, com isso, os ossos esfregam-se contra os ossos causando inflamação nas juntas, principalmente os ossos suportadores de peso que ficam mais sujeitos a adesões e crescimento excessivo de suas extremidades, a saber osteoartrose. O efeito cumulativo de tudo isso se apresenta em forma de rigidez e dor.

O envelhecimento não pode ser evitado, porém seu efeito pode ser diminuído com precauções tomadas com a coluna lombar—um assunto sobre o qual todo mundo deveria estar a par, como o exemplo da higiene dental. Porém, antes de iniciar qualquer cuidado com a coluna lombar, é melhor compreender a mecânica da dor nas costas.

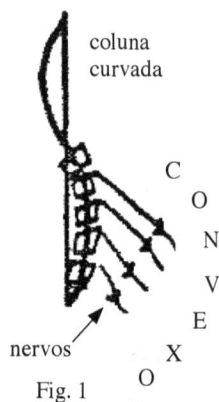

Fig. 1

Se a espinha fosse vista de frente para trás ela seria uma linha reta (fig. 1). Entretanto, em muitas pessoas ela pode ser curvada. As vértebras são os blocos que formam a espinha. Numa espinha curvada, o espaço intervertebral se abre do lado convexo e se estreita do lado côncavo como uma vara entortada. Isso causa uma desigualdade de pressões nas articulações vertebrais predispondo a pessoa à artrose. Observe que, por entre as vértebras, saem nervos espinhais que emergem da medula espinhal. Estes podem ficar comprometidos—esticados demais ou pressionados, aumentando a dor que se irradia da coluna lombar até os membros inferiores, geralmente na parte de trás do membro, o que se refere como dor ciática.

A espinha, vista de lado, tem curvas naturais para frente e para trás (fig. 2).

A coluna lombar é curvada para frente e consite de 5 vértebras (fig. 3). Em cada vértebra se origina um par de processos superior e inferior de cada lado da coluna vertebral. O processo inferior da vértebra superior se articula com o respectivo processo superior da vértebra inferior formando juntas chamadas facetas articulares. A faceta articular é uma junta lubrificada e a constante fricção em sua superfície a predispõe a inflamações.

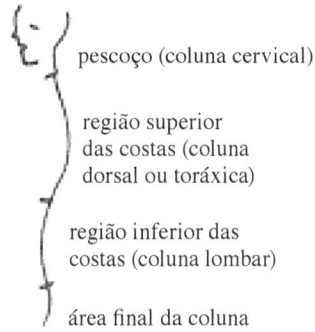

pescoço (coluna cervical)

região superior das costas (coluna dorsal ou toráxica)

região inferior das costas (coluna lombar)

área final da coluna

Fig. 2

Pelo diagrama ao lado, fica fácil visualizar que, se a faceta articular se tornar artrítica ou se houver protusão de um disco comprimido entre as vértebras, as raízes dos nervos que saem do foramen (orifício), conforme ilustrado, podem ficar comprometidas causando a dor ciática além da dor lombar.

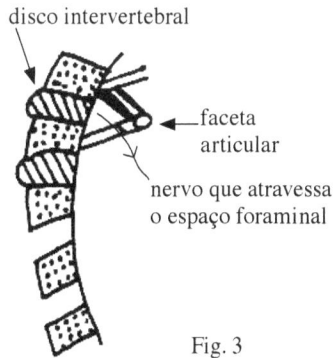

disco intervertebral

faceta articular

nervo que atravessa o espaço foraminal

Fig. 3

Quanto maior a acentuação da curvatura para frente, maior é a probabilidade de inflamação na faceta articular. Quando tal inflamação ocorre (I) a dor aumenta (D), provocando o espasmo (E) dos músculos dos dois lados da espinha (a coluna é como se fosse um entalhe longitudinal entre duas saliências longitudinais dos dois lados

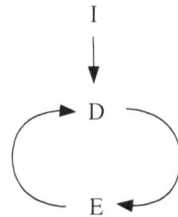

I

D

E

Fig. 4

formadas pelos músculos) o que causa ainda mais dor (fig. 4).

Assim se inicia um ciclo vicioso que pode manifestar-se como uma dor lombar crônica e insuportável, com ou sem agravações agudas e radiação para os membros inferiores.

O que faz aumentar a inclinação da curvatura normal da coluna para frente? (fig. 5)

1. Um aumento da inclinação da curva da parte superior da coluna para trás, uma corcunda (conforme pontilhado na figura).

2. Uma saliência abdominal devido à uma fraqueza na musculatura abnominal, uma barriga grande, gravidez, carregamento de pesos na frente do corpo como fazem as bibliotecárias, isto pressionará a coluna lombar para frente.

diafragma

diafragma pélvico

visão lateral do osso pélvico

inclinação

isquiotibial

Fig. 5

3. Rigidez na musculatura posterior das coxas: estes músculos são ligados desde a parte traseira da região pélvica até a parte traseira do joelho. Se enrigecidos, eles causam uma inclinação da pélvis à qual a coluna está ligada e, consequentemente, uma acentuação da curva para frente.

4. Sapatos de saltos altos: sabe-se que os saltos altos provocam um modo de andar desequilibrado. Isto ocorre porque a parte superior da pélvis se inclina para frente e carrega consigo a parte inferior da coluna.

Muitas outras condições, também, podem causar dor nas costas (ex. Infecções) ou dor ciática (ex. Diabete). Estes assuntos não estão sendo tratados neste artigo o qual se concentra na mecânica normal da dor na coluna lombar. Além disso, sabe-se que estresses mentais e emocionais podem causar dor na coluna. Isto se deve ao estado crônico de tensão muscular e, traduzindo simbolicamente, diríamos carregar um "peso" nas costas ou manter seus próprios problemas para si mesmo.

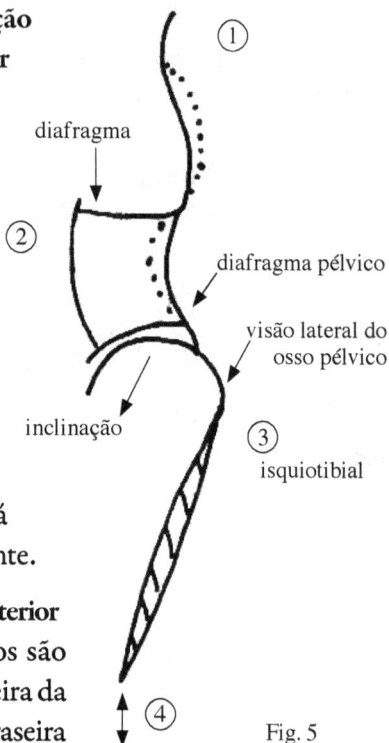

Cuidados com a coluna lombar

Após entender o "por quê" da dor na coluna lombar, fica fácil saber "como" cuidar dela. Entretanto, uma pessoa poderia aplicar esses cuidados mesmo sem entender a mecânica da dor nas costas. Devemos ser realistas com as nossas expectativas. Já que a prevenção total do envelhecimento cronológico da coluna não é possível, podemos apenas retardar os seus efeitos. Portanto, estaríamos, relativamente, prevenindo a dor ou diminuindo a sua amplitude e frequência (fig. 6).

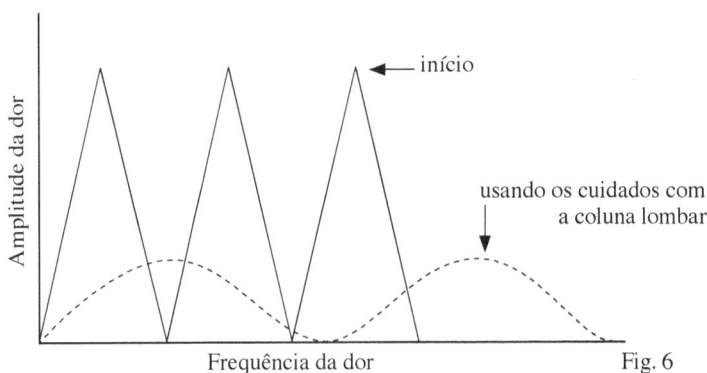

Fig. 6

Se a coluna lombar estiver desalinhada ou curvada quando visualizada de frente para trás ou vice-versa, a correção é feita, simplesmente, aumentando o salto do sapato no lado convexo da curva. Para que você mesmo veja desalinhamentos, fique de pé, sem roupas, com os pés juntos, com os braços esticados para baixo e em frente à um espelho alto. Há, naturalmente, um espaço entre os cotovelos e a cintura. Em uma coluna reta, isto é igual em ambos os lados, mas em uma coluna curvada, o lado convexo é menor e o lado côncavo é maior. Para equilibrar isto, continue aumentando o salto do sapato 1 cm de cada vez do lado convexo (pode-se usar paletas de madeira ou um sapato com a altura do salto diferente) até igualar o espaço. Isto pode ser confirmado pedindo à uma outra pessoa ou um médico para visualizar a sua coluna pelas costas.

A eliminação da acentuação da curvatura para frente na coluna lombar implicaria em fortalecer a musculatura abdominal, relaxar os isquiotibiais, alongar os músculos paraespinhais alongando a coluna para aliviar o espasmo e eliminar ou reduzir o uso de sapatos de saltos altos, todos, especialmente durante episódios de dor. Sapatos com saltos entre ½ a ¾ de uma polegada poderiam ser usados. Se uma pessoa quiser ficar mais alta, seria melhor usar um salto de plataforma.

O ciclo vicioso de inflamação, dor e espasmo precisa ser quebrado usando postura, exercícios, calor, medicamentos e cirurgia (a qual não está sendo tratada aqui). A maioria das dores na coluna lombar pode ser tratada através de métodos conservadores.

Os medicamentos seriam do grupo primordial de anti-inflamatórios, suplementados com remédios para dor quando necessário. Seria melhor tomar os medicamentos com comida e com antiácidos para prevenir irritação na membrana estomacal.

O calor e choque de onda curta diatérmico dados por um fisioterapeuta podem ser aplicados em casa usando uma aplicação de toalha quente e molhada. Cubra as costas com ela e a envolva com um plástico para reter a humidade e o calor. Quando a dor diminuir e os músculos relaxarem, aproveite a oportunidade para praticar exercícios. Saiba que lâmpadas infra-vermelhas não promovem a penetração de calor e, assim sendo, são inúteis.

Postura

Sentado: Não se deve sentar com as costas completamente encostadas na cadeira, como geralmente é ensinado, pois isto aumentará a curvatura frontal da coluna lombar. Sente-se um pouco para frente, com os joelhos elevados, permitindo um relaxamento da coluna lombar. Pode-se cruzar a perna sobre a outra ou apoiar o tornozelo de uma perna sobre o joelho da outra (fig. 7). Ao sentar-se próximo à uma mesa, mova a cadeira para perto da mesa e use o apoio para os pés o qual deve ficar próximo a você (fig. 8). Se não houver este apoio para os pés,

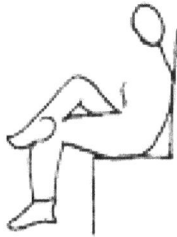
Fig. 7

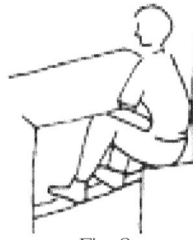
Fig. 8

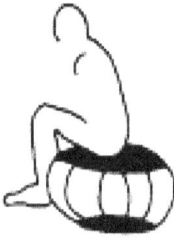
Fig. 9

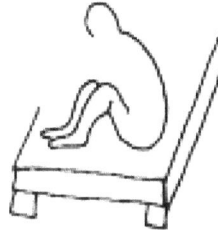
Fig. 10

use uma caixa ou gaveta para descansar os pés. O importante é elevar os joelhos, se possível, acima dos quadris, com isso inclinando a parte inferior da pélvis para frente e forçando a coluna lombar para trás. Em casa, se preferir, pode-se sentar em uma superfície baixa (fig. 9) para que os joelhos fiquem, automaticamente, elevados ou sente-se colocando os pés sobre a superfície também (fig. 10).

Entretanto, em um veículo automotivo, sente-se encostando, completamente, no assento e coloque um pequeno travesseiro na folga que ocorrerá entre a região lombar e a parte superior das costas. Isto aliviará a absorção dos choques ao longo da coluna. Se for dirigir, além do que foi dito acima, mantenha seu assento, confortavelmente, próximo ao painel dos pedais ao ponto de que os joelhos fiquem, suficientemente, elevados.

Deitado: Em uma superfície de madeira, use um colchão firme. Um que seja grosso e de algodão é melhor. Assim, a coluna pode se alinhar sobre ele. Um solo duro é desnecessário, além de ferir as proeminências ósseas.

A coluna não se alinha em um colchão macio. Deitar-se sobre o estômago deve ser evitado já que a coluna lombar fica inclinada para trás e com uma curva para frente. Se for deitar de barriga

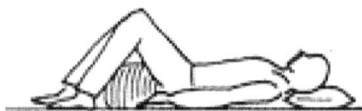

Fig. 11

para cima, flexione os joelhos, apoie a sola
dos pés sobre a cama e use um travesseiro
de apoio ou duas almofadas debaixo dos
joelhos para sustentação. Essa postura deixa a
coluna lombar reta sobre a cama (fig. 11). Se for
deitar de lado, (caso esteja de barriga cheia, é mais
confortável deitar sobre o lado esquerdo, assim o
estômago recebe sustentação) flexione a bacia e os
joelhos, leve-os em direção ao peito, podendo um
estar mais elevado que o outro (fig. 12).

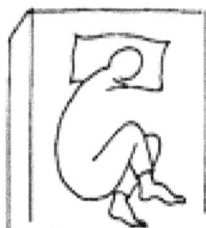

Fig. 12

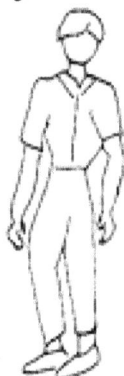

Em pé: Intermitentemente, sentar-se apro-
priadamente ou curvar-se para frente e supender o
dorso ligeiramente, quando possível, requer muito
esforço da coluna. Ao ficar de pé com as duas pernas esticadas,
a pélvis se mantém em uma posição travada. A todo momento,
pode-se destravá-la e o que ajuda é flexionar um joelho um
pouco e, levemente, inclinar a pélvis para o lado oposto. (fig. 13).

Fig. 13

Trabalhar de pé, como cozinhar, passar roupas, etc., pode
ser destrutivo para a coluna lombar. Os "prós" e os "contra" estão
ilustrados (fig. 14). Mantenha seu corpo próximo ao balcão de
trabalho. Ter um espaço para encaixar os pés debaixo do balcão
de trabalho, ajuda. Use um apoio para colocar debaixo do pé e,
de tempo em tempo, troque um pé pelo outro alternadamente.

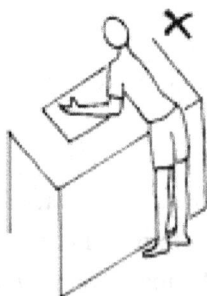
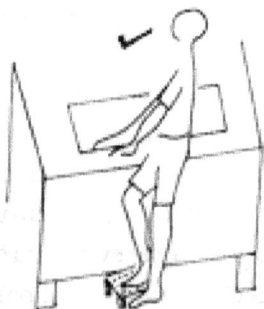

Fig. 14

Caminhar: De novo, intermitentemente sentar-se ou curvar-se para frente e suspender seu dorso ligeiramente é muito bom.

Levantar peso: A coluna fica no seu ponto mais fraco se estiver em uma posição inclinada e curvada para frente. Imagine bloquinhos de brinquedo de criança colocados, exatamente, um sobre o outro na posição vertical. Um toque no topo deles não irá derrubá-los. Entretanto, se forem colocados em posição curvada, ao serem tocados, eles cairíam facilmente.

Quando se carrega pesos na frente do corpo com as pernas mais ou menos esticadas e curva-se a coluna para frente, o fulcro fica na coluna e o peso fica distante, o que não promove nenhuma vantagem mecânica, forçando a coluna. Sempre que possível, mantenha o peso próximo a lateral de seu corpo. Flexione as pernas, mantenha a coluna, relativamente, reta e, ao esticar as pernas, use os músculos fortalecidos para ajudar a levantar o peso (fig. 15).

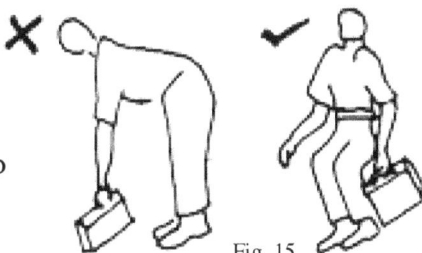

Fig. 15

Exercícios

Juntamente à uma boa postura, estes promovem o suporte da coluna lombar. Os exercícios têm o propósito de alongar os músculos paraespinhais espasmódicos, fortalecer a musculatura abdominal, relaxar os isquiotibiais, eliminar adesões nas juntas sinoviais e ajudar a auto-manipulação da coluna.

Exercícios na posição em pé

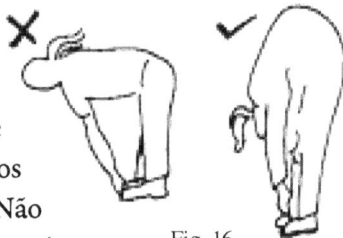

Fig. 16

1. **Tocar os dedos dos pés:** Junte os pés. Tente tocar os dedos dos pés curvando-se para frente. Não comece a inclinar o dorso a partir dos quadris e curve-se. Cuidado ao flexionar a coluna, tente manter a cabeça próxima ao peito curvando uma vértebra

de cada vez (fig. 16). Alcançar os dedos dos pés ou o solo não é o objetivo, mas tente curvar-se para frente o máximo que conseguir. Evite curvar-se bruscamente para frente. No entanto, levantar-se ligeiramente é bom. Exalar ajuda durante o movimento de flexão para baixo.

2. **Virar e girar:** os pés afastados um do outro à distância de 0,45 m, as mãos nos quadris, vire o máximo para a esquerda (fig. 17). Então, ligeiramente, volte à posição inicial e, suavemente, gire até o máximo de novo. Gire duas vezes. Volte à posição inicial. Agora, vire e repita a mesma manobra para a direita. Se tiver problemas com os joelhos, seria melhor praticar este exercício sentado bem na beira de uma cadeira sem braços ou de uma cama. Isto evitará torcer o joelho.

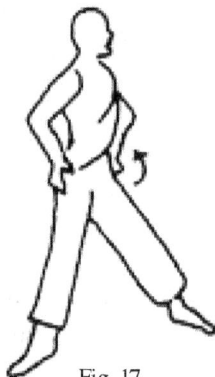

Fig. 17

3. **Tocar os dedos de um dos pés com a mão contrária àquele lado:** os pés bem afastados. Com os dedos da mão direita, tente tocar os dedos do pé do lado esquerdo (fig. 18). Volte à posição inicial. Agora, o contrário.

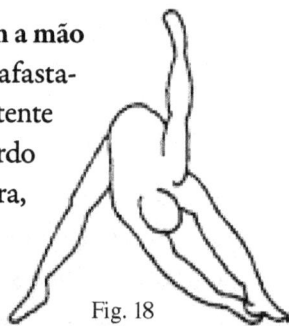

4. **Alternar o toque nos dedos dos pés e calcanhar:** os pés bem afastados.

Fig. 18

Com os dedos da mão esquerda, tente tocar os dedos do pé deste mesmo lado. Volte à posição inicial. Agora, tente alcançar o calcanhar direito com os dedos da mão direita (fig. 19). Volte à posição inicial. Agora, o contrário.

5. **Flexão lateral:** os pés bem afastados. Os braços esticados para os lados. Flexione para o lado esquerdo levando o braço esquerdo ao lado da perna esquerda. Estique o braço direito para cima e vire a cabeça na mesma direção (fig. 20). Volte à posição inicial. Repita isto com o lado direito.

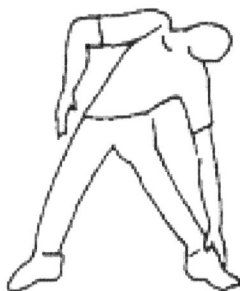

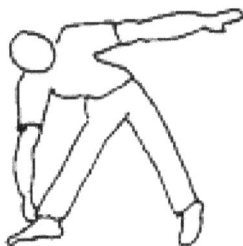

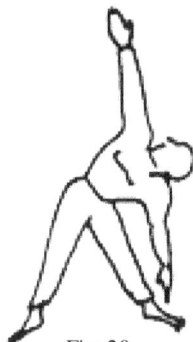

Fig. 19   Fig. 20

6. Chutar: Dê um ou dois passos para frente e eleve a perna esquerda para cima para tocar os dedos da mão esquerda que deve manter-se esticada para frente na altura do seu ombro (fig. 21). Cuidado para não escorregar ou cair para trás, evitando piso ou calçados escorregadios. Agora, repita com o lado direito.

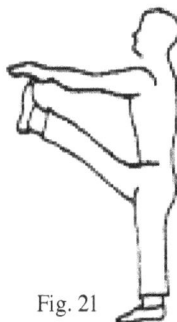

Fig. 21

Exercícios em decúbito dorsal:

(em uma superfície firme ou dura, por exemplo, em cima de uma coberta sobre o solo)

7. Mãos para trás da cabeça. Junte os pés. Estenda as pernas para frente. Inspire e segure o fôlego. Eleve os pés algumas polegadas do solo até que haja um esforço máximo no meio de seu abdômen, segure esta posição contando até dez (talvez você tenha que treinar um pouco, até que consiga manter esta posição na contagem até dez) depois abaixe os pés (fig. 22).

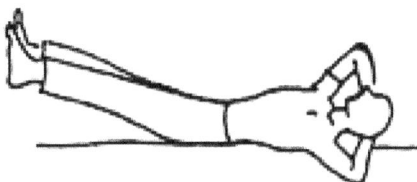

Fig. 22

8. Repita o exercício acima com os pés bem afastados. O esforço será sentido, principalmente, na região baixa e lateral do abdômen.

9. Deite de barriga para cima com os braços para baixo ao lado do corpo. Flexione o quadril e o joelho esquerdo abraçando-o com as mãos bem abaixo dele. Traga-o até o seu ombro direito, o qual pode se curvar para frente também. Mantenha a perna direita estendida (fig. 23). Expirar ajuda. Repita isto com o lado oposto.

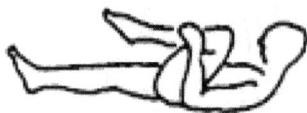

Fig. 23

10. Deite de barriga para cima e com os braços esticados acima da cabeça. Levante o dorso e tente alcançar os dedos dos pés (fig. 24). Expirar ajuda. Se você não conseguir levantar seu dorso, peça a alguém para segurar as suas pernas ou apoie seus dedos dos pés debaixo de um móvel pesado, como uma cômoda, para lhe ajudar. Se você não conseguir alcançar os seus dedos dos pés, segure a parte das pernas que você conseguir alcançar e empurre seu dorso para baixo como se fosse colocar a sua cabeça entre as pernas.

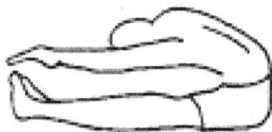

Fig. 24

Cada um dos exercícios acima devem ser feitos três vezes. Demora em torno de 7 minutos. Geralmente, uma vez por dia é o suficiente. Se houver dor, recomenda-se duas vezes ao dia.

Saiba que alongar a coluna para frente ajuda a aumentar o espaço do canal medular nas vértebras, através do qual a medula espinhal emerge do cérebro. Também, aumenta o espaço foraminal o que alivia a compressão dos nervos. Isto é mais um benefício para o tratamento de dores neurais que se irradiam na coluna.

Cuidado. Muitas outras condicões também podem aumentar a dor da coluna lombar ou a dor ciática. Tais condições devem ser investigadas e eliminadas, na maioria das vezes, através de exames sanguíneos e radiografias. Entretanto, a maioria das dores nas costas se encaixam na categoria do fenômeno de esforço e podem ser tratadas usando os cuidados com a coluna lombar.

Por fim, estresses psicológicos precisam ser tratados através de técnicas de relaxamento e do conhecimento da arte de viver.

Low Back Pain and Low Back Care

Aviso:

O conteúdo deste livro é direcionado para a maioria dos casos de lombalgia mecânica e não para infecções, tumores, etc. Por favor, consulte um médico para descobrir a causa da sua dor nas costas. O autor, os tradutores e a editora não se responsabilizam por qualquer dano que possa surgir após a utilização do conteúdo deste livro (mesmo sabendo que nenhum tenha ocorrido).

www.ingramcontent.com/pod-product-compliance
Lightning Source LLC
Chambersburg PA
CBHW050600280326
41933CB00011B/1918